Winning
the
Losing
Battle

Eda J. LeShan

Thomas Y. Crowell, Publishers

ESTABLISHED 1834, NEW YORK

Winning the Losing Battle

Why I Will Never Be Fat Again

Designer: Leslie Phillips

LIBRARY OF CONGRESS CATALOGING IN PUBLICATION DATA
LeShan, Eda J.
  Winning the losing battle.

  1. Reducing—Psychological aspects. I. Title.
RM222.2.L426   1979   613.2'5'019   79–7093
ISBN 0–690–01845–2

  80 81 82 83 10 9 8 7 6 5

Contents

Acknowledgments

By this time there have been so many people who helped me to lose weight and write the book that all I can do is list those very special people who gave the most support in one way or another.

First of all, my deepest thanks to the entire medical and administrative staff at the Duke University Private Diagnostic Clinic, who could not have been kinder or more encouraging. And then, for reasons they each know best: Susie and Bil Baird, Grace Bechtold, Jean Lee Brandman, Deborah and Angela Cruser, Barbara Cullum, Arnold Dolin, Edith Engel, Richard Grossman, Sylvia Halpern, Wendy Jackson, Marc Jaffe, Maria Janis, Bev Kennedy, Miriam Koenig, Florence Miale, Lee Polk, Barbara Ratliff, David Reuther, Squire Rushnell, Natalie Stein, Linda Tolpel, and Phyllis Wender.

1

The Agony
of Being Fat–
the Terror
of Being Thin

It's over—it's really been over for a long time now. I started not being fat in January 1977, at the age of fifty-four, having struggled with various degrees of obesity since I was seven or eight. I will never be fat again.

I have been sitting at my desk in my summer home on Cape Cod, thinking about this remarkable fact of my life. It is raining and I face a picture window that overlooks a lake. In the window I see a reflection of the fire in the fireplace behind me—and dimly I see the reflection of a woman sitting at a typewriter. She startles me; I have trouble seeing she is *me*. And yet I know her very well—we have been through a great deal together. She is sixty-five pounds lighter than she was that January; I feel a sense of wonder and thanksgiving. I am a formerly fat person who will never be fat again. It is the most surprising and miraculous thing I know about myself—but there was no miracle.

As millions of other people do, I used to buy every diet book, try every new diet, work endlessly with doctors, lose weight— and always gain it all back again (as do 90 to 95 percent of all the other people who try to lose weight). *Except this time.* What I discovered is that there is no way to *stay* thin unless one is psychologically ready before the dieting ever begins, and that being ready requires confronting a terror of being thin. I finally figured out that as agonizing as it may be to be overweight, it is nothing compared to the anxiety of changing from a fat person to a thin one.

After years of struggling to solve the mystery of why I always gained back whatever weight I might successfully lose, I discovered that I was actually terrified of being thin. I now believe that this is true for most overweight people. Each new diet is begun in a state of great ambivalence, which undermines our progress and dooms us to eventual failure.

I worked long and hard on preparing myself, and what I learned is this: No permanent weight loss can take place until there has been a profound change in one's attitudes and feelings about oneself. By the time I actually began to diet, I thought I had figured out exactly how to do it. And since I had decided to write a book about my experiences in getting ready to be thin, I started keeping a daily journal of the dieting process.

When I began to write the book, I expected to focus almost entirely on the critical period *before* a diet is undertaken. But what I discovered was that no matter how well I may have prepared myself to lose weight, the process itself involved constant new adjustments and insights. The period *during* the dieting was as important as the preparation. And once I had lost the weight, I realized there was still more to learn, more need for change; *after* the period of dieting I had to come to terms with a new self.

There is an awful impatience these days with anything that takes time. We want to give one primal scream and be cured! One weekend of self-revelation and a total personality change!

But there are no shortcuts, no panaceas that will effectively produce long-term results. The only way to lose weight and keep it off is to deal with the complexity, the subtlety, the depth of our feelings.

For me, the first stage of getting ready to lose weight permanently involved examining and conquering my irrational terror of being thin, of changing from a fat person to a thin one. The second stage involved becoming so sensitized to my own needs, both physiological and psychological, that I could search for and find the diet best suited to me individually. The third stage (and this came as a total surprise when it happened) was to go through a time for grief and mourning for the fat self I was giving up.

In the course of many years of psychotherapy, I wrote copious notes concerning that part of my self—discoveries having to do with being overweight. During the period of dieting—and all through the writing of this book—I have kept a daily journal about what I was feeling, how I was behaving. It has been a process in which both figuratively and literally I have peeled away layer after layer of myself, and learned to understand more and more.

I lived for three and a half months with some three hundred fat people under the supervision of Dr. Walter Kempner on the Rice Diet program at the Duke University Medical Center in Durham, North Carolina. My fellow patients ranged in age from sixteen to the mid seventies, came from all parts of the country, from all walks of life, with widely differing medical problems and individual life experiences. The large majority were women. More fat women than fat men seem to be able to deal with their obesity—but of course the fact that the program requires one to leave home for a period of time could certainly have been a factor in the proportion of men in the program, since men still tend to be the major wage earners in most families.

While living in Durham, I learned a great deal about all the rich variation of distinct personal differences, but I was also able to verify my own judgments by the universality of so many of our feelings and experiences. On the surface we may have seemed to be very different, but psychologically we were brothers and sisters in our shared suffering.

I have given a good deal of thought to how best to make use of the marvelous insights and the tender humanity of my "fellow inmates" in Durham, without violating their privacy and without confusing the issues they raised. What I have done is to draw on the different qualities and problems of these people to invent a cast of characters. Although none of my characters could be identified as one of the actual patients, I have tried to make each person consistent and real, inventing nothing that didn't actually happen.

It would be impossible for me to describe my own experience without referring to the diet that finally "worked" for me. I urge you—I plead with you—not to assume that it is the right diet for you. I believe that in all matters of medical treatment and care, every individual has his or her own idiosyncratic reactions. I believe we have to find the method, the style, that suits each of us best, and fortunately there is an infinite variety of programs now available to fulfill every individual's unique requirements. Some of you will think that my route would also suit you; if that's the case, explore it. But I can't stress too strongly that a diet cannot work unless it is specifically designed to fit the individual.

What I am concerned with, far more than the question of any specific diet, is to try to remove the secrecy of our pain and suffering, to reveal our terrible hurts, fears, self-condemnation. That is the beginning of getting ready to diet and stay thin. What I propose is that you follow me through my personal odyssey, and if it makes sense to you, that you begin to use it as a guideline for your own explorations. I would not have bothered to write this book if I did not believe that had someone given me such a book twenty or thirty years ago I could have lost weight and kept it off then.

I believe that what I went through will strike a chord of recognition in most other fat people. I think what I learned can be helpful to others. If you are willing to begin to examine your own life and to work at changing and growing, with honesty and courage, it is possible for you to lose weight and to keep it off. I offer you my companionship in that struggle. I cannot predict where you will go or how, precisely, you will do it. It is ultimately an individual process, to which you will have to bring your own special and unique background, personality, needs and dreams. But we do share many similarities—of that I am absolutely convinced. I think I know much of your pain; I know the pitfalls and the terrors. I think I can help. Please—*do not start dieting* until you have finished this book. No cheating! It is about *getting ready*. I did. So can you. Let us begin.

The Agony of Being Fat

Every time I see a fat person, I know that in some ways he or she wants to die; obesity is, after all, a slow form of suicide. Some of us cry a lot, others laugh enough to reinforce the myth that we are a jolly group—but whatever we do, it is agony to be fat.

Many years ago, trying desperately to diet, I wrote in my diary:

> I'm gripped by this terrible compulsion. I can't stop eating. I feel as if there is no limit; I could walk into a candy store and eat everything on the shelves. I'm filled with horror and self-disgust. I'm destroying my life. When I lie down I can feel a throbbing in my head—all over my body sometimes—I know I may be giving myself high blood pressure or diabetes or an assortment of other dangerous diseases.

Why am I so totally undisciplined, so stupid, so powerless?
I despise myself.

Even when we diet, we play the game. Some eat less than
they are supposed to, get weak and tired and start overeating
again, while others eat more than they are supposed to. I've
never met anyone on a diet who didn't spend a good deal of
time figuring out when and how to cheat. In Durham we all
knew that if we weren't out ourselves, the nights were full of
prowlers, looking for pizzas and cheeseburgers and french fries.
On the surface it looks as if we are giving ourselves gifts, but
just the reverse is true. We cannot stop punishing ourselves
for being fat and so we get fatter.

Shortly after arriving in Durham, I wrote in my journal:

> There was a woman at our table at lunch today who weighs
> three hundred pounds. She was here for nine months and
> then again for six months, over the past couple of years.
> Her father is a cardiologist and he told her, "You'll be dead
> in six months if you don't lose weight." She laughed and
> said, "So why am I back here? I'm just a compulsive eater—
> I like food." She has diabetes and she told us it improved
> very dramatically as long as she stayed on the diet. Now
> she's back on insulin. "I guess I must have gotten used to
> the injections—maybe I missed them." More loud laughter.
> "Well, maybe this time I'll be a good girl." *Be a good girl.*
> Self-hatred and wanting to please others. That's the theme,
> over and over again.

On another morning I wrote: "Ruth came in to the Rice House
[where we had our meals and daily checkups], took her coat
off and said, "Well, I guess I gotta weigh this disgusting body.'"

The Theory-of-the-Month Club

New "wonder ways" for losing weight are about as plentiful
as theories about why we get fat in the first place—and yet

the truth is we still know very little about obesity. Fatness is a very complex subject involving cultural attitudes, heredity, physiology and human emotions. It's impossible to tell where one factor begins and another ends, or how each influences the other.

Heredity undoubtedly plays a role in obesity, but no one knows for sure just how. There seem to be family tendencies. Some people can eat like horses and maintain the same weight all their adult lives, while others who are quite careful of what they eat may struggle constantly with weight problems. It is impossible to arrive at any clear answer because family eating patterns are inextricably interwoven with hereditary tendencies.

There is undoubtedly some relation between a tendency to gain weight and how much we exercise. There seems to be some logic to the notion that if we never move, we can't burn up enough calories, and in general, very active people are not usually overweight. But we all know *very lazy* skinny people too.

There is little, if any, agreement about the complex variables affecting the biochemical aspects of obesity. Until quite recently, any obese person who blamed her overweight on physical causes was made to feel guilty and ashamed by most of the medical profession. But this attitude has begun to change as new concepts and theories arise from continuing research. We have been hearing more and more in the last few years about "fat cells." In 1971 Dr. Jerome Knittle, a researcher at the National Institutes of Health, reported that the child who is going to be obese can be identified at the age of two years, by ascertaining with considerable accuracy the number of fat cells he has.

Obese people have a higher number of fat cells than the non-obese, and those cells are generally bigger as well. Apparently, fat babies grow up into fat adults because of cellular structure which causes an abnormal number of fat cells to "crave" to return to their former size when normal eating is resumed after dieting.

Those of us who have been fat for many years know instinctively that there are other factors that remain to be investigated, such as individual differences. Different foods affect each person differently at different times, and some foods make us much hungrier than other foods. Maybe, when we are much too old and decrepit to care anymore, there will be a little white pill you can take in the morning, confident that by the next day you will have lost a pound or two!

The strange complexities of food and body chemistry came up for discussion many times while I was in Durham. I often had the feeling that if researchers would only *listen* to the crazy, intuitive reactions of fat people, they might learn a good deal. For example, I *know* that the crucial reason the Rice Diet worked for me was the drastic cutting out of salt from my diet. I felt better than I'd felt in years—but even more important, I stopped craving sweets. I have been unable to find a consistent or satisfactory answer for this phenomenon.

During the months on the Rice Diet, I was very aware of how little we still know about it all. Helpful as the program was to me and to many others—for a variety of medical problems—I often had the feeling that it must be similar to the programs that were designed for victims of tuberculosis fifty years ago. All kinds of elaborate and seemingly whimsical approaches were used—years of isolation and bed rest, sleeping on open porches in freezing weather in some mountaintop sanitarium. Who then could have believed that TB would someday be cured by a drug that could be taken while one continued to lead a normal life? Fifty years from now, our current approaches to obesity will probably seem just as archaic.

But for those of us alive and fat today, that is no help. Unfortunately, whatever the complex causes of our problem, once we become obese we tend to learn very quickly to use food to "solve" all the normal problems of life—for the moment. Nothing hurts so much that it can't be soothed by a piece of chocolate cake, by a hamburger and french fries and a malted. For short periods of time we feel comforted, happy. We run for the cookie jar to assuage feelings of jealousy, anxiety, boredom, restlessness, anger, sadness, fear, frustration and depression. We drown our sorrows in quarts of ice cream. But following such moments of gratification there is a terrible aftermath of deep gloom and an intense feeling of self-contempt. Compulsive overeating takes on a life of its own, totally unrelated to hunger; it becomes an instantaneous response to every emotional problem.

Since medical science does not yet offer us any truly satisfactory answers, what are our options at this point? Well, the answer I have arrived at is that we use the best information we can possibly get about nutrition and biology—and then we have to accept the fact that if we are going to lose weight and keep it off, we will have to focus most of our attention on the psychological aspects of obesity. We know a good deal about that. And furthermore, dieting itself involves so much self-denial, such will power, that we really have no choice but to deal with the emotional torment involved.

The Getting-Ready Theory

One thing I am certain about—until you have reached a certain level of readiness, it is pointless to go on a diet, because eventually you are bound to gain back the weight you lose.

In the course of my long struggle, I tried to deal with every possible aspect of my problem—my heredity, my childhood and adolescence, my adulthood. By the time I finally found the right diet and was able to stick to it, I had discovered that none of all this groundwork could pay off—I couldn't really be ready—*until I had learned to love myself fat.* I had identified the enemy—and the enemy was *me.* Ultimately, readiness is a personal affirmation; not the fear of dying, not shame or guilt, but finding oneself lovable—and worthy of care.

I began to understand this several years before I finally dieted successfully. I was in my first exercise class at a Florida diet spa. There I was in a bright-red sweat suit, clumsily trying to touch my toes without bending my knees. It was a situation that would once have caused me terrible embarrassment and mortification. What had happened that had made it possible for me to be there? What had changed that made it possible for me to do some of the exercises and refuse to do others, or to quit in the middle if it got to be too much? How had I found the courage necessary to be able to stand in the midst of mostly agile and slender women who were doing the exercises beautifully—and not feel the slightest urge to drown feelings of overwhelming self-hatred in a five-pound box of chocolates?

It took me two days to realize that most people hate their bodies, whatever they look like objectively. No one was the least bit interested in my body—*I* was the interested party. And I was *somebody;* I mattered to me. That was all that was important—that I had finally cared enough, been proud enough, to come for needed help. If I was fat and out of shape, that was just about *the only thing that was seriously wrong with me!* And it was a solvable problem—far easier than if I'd been stupid or mean or untalented or irresponsible!

It was not the repeated nightmare of my childhood in which people laughed at me or made fun of me. I felt marvelous! I was a grown woman of some accomplishment. I was a loved woman and I was making a choice, without shame, without anger at myself.

This was an important first step in the process of changing. At that time I lost about ten pounds in ten days. I was beginning to care for myself. It was a first step in respect and concern for my physical well-being. I was allowing myself to realize I had only this one body to see me through all my years. I could not go on abusing myself indefinitely without serious consequences. Now that I was over fifty years old, feeling well was no longer something I could take for granted. It was time to be more loving toward myself.

Whatever other factors may be involved, we get fat and stay fat primarily because we hate ourselves. *What we cannot deny ourselves is food; what we continually deny ourselves is self-love.* How did we get that way? Until we know why this happens to us, until we can deal with whatever our personal demons may be, it is almost impossible to change our behavior toward ourselves. Obesity is one of the ways we have chosen to torment ourselves for what we unconsciously, irrationally presume to be our terrible and unbearable sins. The reason we diet but never get thin is that we have tried to solve the problem without fully understanding the agonizing pain we carry with us—a far more terrible burden than our extra weight.

In the course of the past twenty to twenty-five years, I have been my own detective—or explorer—slowly peeling away layer after layer of mostly forgotten or fully unconscious reasons why I needed to have some way of punishing myself, some way of closing myself off from the fullest expression of selfhood.

I discovered, for example, that on one level, the extra weight was a kind of armor—a way of keeping people *out.* There were too many demands, too many expectations, and I wanted so much to be a good girl and please my parents. I once dreamed of myself as an armadillo, encased in an inpenetrable leathery shield. On another level, food served to make me sleepy, lethargic. I sometimes dreamed of myself as a hippopotamus, lying in a mud puddle in the sun. Eating too much, being fat, was a way of controlling libidinal drives that frightened me. I was afraid to deal with the energy that smoldered within. At one time, being fat also represented a fantasy of being pregnant. Being fat meant being strong and healthy too. I had a feeling that if I got thin I might die. (How many of us were told as children that if we didn't eat we would never grow up, would

get very sick?) And—perhaps most fundamentally—it was a re-
fusal to give myself the gift of what I considered to be physical
attractiveness.

As I explored the many dark alleys of my own feelings and
experiences and compared them to those of others, I found the
following to be the crucial issues in our inability to lose weight
permanently:

1. We share a special kind of guilt: We are usually people who
have tried quite desperately to please others—first our parents,
then our spouses, children, bosses, co-workers, friends, relatives
and neighbors. By the time we are fat adults, we are angry at
ourselves for having spent so much of our lives in pursuit of
this empty, meaningless quest, this trying to please everyone
but ourselves. We know, at some deep level of consciousness,
that we have sold out, that we are not who we want and need
to be. The shame and guilt are so profound that self-destruction
seems inevitable.

We are also likely to be people who are in terror of facing
the possibility that maybe we are quite special. This was something about which I tormented myself most of my life, and
hid beneath layers and layers of fat—and now I cannot understand why. What is so terrible about *not being ordinary?*

All the years of self-exploration seemed finally to culminate
in this "terrifying" fact that I was born with special gifts and
needed to use them. It is hard to explain why that was a problem;
after all, my parents felt I was special, and many teachers re-
marked on my talents, and I had friends who felt I was special.
I even behaved as if I was special—but only within carefully
circumscribed limits.

. Some children are born with more fire, more vitality, more
creativity, more gifts, than others. When you have all that going
for you as a child, you are likely to move in one of two directions.
Chances are that those qualities can make you a rebel, an oddball
among your peers, and with parents and other adults. You can

endure the pain of being different and get into a lot of trouble as a kid—or you can do everything possible to hide your talents and masquerade as a regular, average sort of person.

A few years ago I met a schoolmate I hadn't seen since 1940, when we graduated from high school. She was much "smarter"— got A's in everything. I assumed that when we were grown up she would be a great success and I would be a failure. I now know I "arranged" things that way: I had such anxiety attacks that I was bound to fail exams; I was so preoccupied with the struggle not to rebel and yet to still fight to be myself that I had no energy for concentrating on difficult subjects. Well, Helen turned out to be one of the most boring women I have ever met! We had nothing to say to each other. We disliked each other on sight. She said she had read some of my books and articles and added, "It doesn't surprise me that you turned out to be such a radical person." When I showed obvious surprise, she added, "We all knew you were different from us, that sooner or later you'd be the one to rock the boat." Apparently, my secret was not as well kept as I had thought. Many of us have to face the fact that we wanted to be rebels—and had the necessary talents to be ahead of our contemporaries, to be leaders—but we were afraid that this would make us unlovable; we wanted desperately to *please*, but not to make waves. There is nothing like a lot of fat to suppress such potential. I wrote about this in Durham, in my journal:

There were five of us on the porch after lunch today. Sylvia began to talk about herself—she's always seen herself as a loser. The other three women leaned forward in their chairs. They all said that they had thought of themselves as passive, dull people without much talent. I asked them if they had ever had dreams for themselves that were different from what they were actually doing. We began sharing the ways in which we had tried so hard to be good, to please other people, do what was expected of us, measure up to someone else's expectations. Joan said, "You know what we're saying? Not a single one of us started out thinking it would be all right to be ourselves!" Claire got very excited. She said, "First I tried to satisfy my parents. Then I got married and worked my ass off putting my husband through law school. When he left me because I was getting fatter, I found a guy who was going into bankruptcy. He owned a diner and I worked my ass off helping him get back on his feet. Then he was finished with me. Each time I felt as if I deserved what I got—even though I was doing exactly what they wanted me to do. Why was that?" Edith answered her: "It's a self-fulfilling prophecy; if you feel like a piece of shit, people treat you as if you are."

2. *We hate ourselves:* Of course, self-hatred doesn't make us unique at all! But the problem is that we cannot lose weight permanently until we are capable of loving ourselves fat. This is true even of people who are just slightly overweight and want to lose a few pounds. While I was in Durham, a friend phoned me from New York, and I wrote about our conversation in my diary:

> She said, "Oh, god, I *know* how you must feel. I feel *so fat.* I can't *stand* it!" She is five feet six and weighs 127 pounds. Unless she weighs under 122, she feels terribly fat. My first instinct was to scream at her in fury—but then it occurred to me that fat people have a lot to learn from thin people who *think* they are fat!

What in the world could possibly make a slender, well-proportioned, attractive young woman think of herself as fat? What does fat mean to her? In our culture, fat and ugly are synonymous. Betty was telling me that she thinks she is ugly. She needs to *think* of herself as fat for very much the same reasons some of us *are* fat. It is a way of feeling that one is no damned good.

Every time we go on a diet and lose weight, people begin

to tell us how well we look; we feel wonderful; we move more easily; we don't get out of breath; we begin to look at the advertisements for fashionable clothes. All this appears on the surface to be making us happy, but in truth it becomes increasingly unbearable. Who are we, to be so happy? It is not to be endured. What I discovered finally, after all the years of struggle, was that I was terrified of being thin because then, for sure, I would have to stop hating myself.

By the time I went to Durham I believed—to my utter astonishment—that I was beautiful and lovable. I continued to have momentary periods of self-dislike—and still do and probably always will—but now I recognize the pattern more quickly and can control it to a much greater extent. Actually, for at least a year before I went on the diet, I had been able to accept my basic lovableness without shame or terror.

3. There is a variety of reasons why we are terrified of being thin: Soon after I arrived in Durham, I wrote in my journal:

> I'm terrified that something will happen to Larry because I can't be allowed to be thin and happily married too. I will be punished if I am too happy. I warded off evil by being fat. It was the price I paid for my good fortune in other aspects of my life.

That is an all too human irrational fear of tempting the gods. I learned that all my terrors were equally irrational fantasies. Like most children, I was exhorted to eat so that I would grow up to be big and strong; not eating might make me puny and weak—and apparently, it had even occurred to me as a child that I might disappear completely.

Another irrational terror from early childhood was that if I didn't eat I would lose love. Here is an entry from my diary after I had tried hypnosis as an aid to dieting:

> I wasn't a very good subject, and I felt both disappointment and relief. I could never have gone to see Dr. D. if I hadn't

reached a point of desperation—and yet, somehow, there is still such a terror of losing something more than just the extra weight—of losing something precious. I think it is because I equate food with love. I can remember sitting at the dining room table at my grandfather's house, feeling so happy, so safe; everyone I loved was there, and the enjoyment of eating together was so important.

I think I have always been afraid that if I got thin and stopped eating too much, these happy memories of childhood would disappear. In fact, to deny the pleasure afforded by food would be to deliberately wipe out the memories of childhood—it would be a kind of *disloyalty*.

One of our most common fantasies—and the source of much terror—is that if we get thin we will lose all control over our libidinal drives. This subject appears and reappears through my Durham journal:

Martha called today. She has gained ten pounds in the last couple of months and she's in a panic. She must weigh all of 125 now! I find it so hard to understand the fat complex of so many really skinny people. Martha is forever on a diet—absolutely hysterical if she gains a quarter of a pound. I think today I finally figured it out. As long as she thinks she's fat ("ugly") she feels as safe as I do; she, too, will be a "good girl." If she ever thought of herself as thin, *she* would be a "bad girl" too! We had a hilarious discussion about our fantasies. After she loses ten pounds and I lose another twenty-five, we are going to go out and buy ourselves dresses with lots of feathers and sequins, and hustle on Eighth Avenue—just for a few days, to get rid of this particular neurosis. "Let's *do* it and get it *over* with!" she said. After much hysterical laughing, I said, "But, Martha, you're thin now, and you're not a whore." "Don't confuse me with reality," she replied, and hung up!

A second entry:

> Joan told me today, "The trouble with me is that under
> all the blubber, I was always a sensual person. I felt I had
> something to hide—I had to insulate myself. It worked quite
> well. Once in a while there would be some perceptive male
> who would see hidden possibilities through the wall of flesh,
> and increase my anxiety level (and fantasy life) incredibly,
> but I would always eat my way back to safety. I felt that
> there was something wrong with me—that I was bad. What
> could have happened? Was I 'playing doctor' with a little
> boy? Did they find me masturbating and enjoying it? God
> knows. At any rate, I'm still scared."

Somewhere along the way (mostly during adolescence), many
of us decided that libidinal feelings were too dangerous and
needed to be denied and repressed. As a result, we have never
learned that one can have feelings and still control them—still
make choices. We never let ourselves find that out.

Before we are ready to lose weight, we have to learn that
we can choose what we do or don't do. Getting thin did not
turn me into a wanton woman! I make choices all the time—
and they reflect my basic attitudes toward life and relationships.
I didn't stop thinking and evaluating because I lost weight; and
under all that fat was no amoral creature of unbridled passions,
but a perfectly sound person capable of discipline and responsible self-control.

Another kind of terror is the fear of becoming narcissistic,
egocentric or selfish. During the period when I was dieting,
I'd get angry every time a friend said, "I want to go shopping
with you when you're thin." I felt superior to people who spent
half their lives shopping. Now I know that in some ways I
envied them. When a friend said she wanted to go to a special
discount store with me after I'd gotten thinner, I yelled at her,
"I'm changing my *size*, not my *personality!*" Even when I said

that, I wondered if it was true. I had this rigid formula: One
who goes shopping a lot is a superficial person; one who, like
me, hates shopping and spends very little time in self-adornment
is a good person, a "contributor to society," a worthy human
being. It was what I call my Eleanor Roosevelt complex.

I became acutely aware of the underlying fear after I had
lost forty pounds in Durham:

> Yesterday I bought myself a pair of slacks and two new
> blouses, to celebrate this landmark. I had planned to treat
> myself to a piece of fried chicken—how marvelous it was
> to realize I wanted the clothes much more! The slacks were
> size 16, the blouses size 14. I could not believe it and asked
> the saleslady two or three times if they could possibly be
> mislabeled, since I'd left New York wearing a 20½. I did
> not recognize the woman in the mirror—she seemed to be
> a total stranger. I felt frightened and depressed . . . but
> this morning I had a marvelous time.
>
> I came downstairs to take the bus to breakfast (it was
> raining very hard), and as I came into the lobby of our
> motel everyone began whistling and cheering. It was *heaven.*
> They all said I looked sensational, and suddenly I found
> myself saying, "This is just the beginning, folks! From now
> on, I'm going to spend money on clothes, I'm going to spend
> half my life looking in mirrors, I'm going to buy makeup
> and jewelry. It's my time, world. Step aside everybody—
> Eda's not taking care of anyone anymore!"
>
> It was as if I had set off fireworks. Everybody began chant-
> ing, shouting and cheering. I hadn't realized what I was
> doing, but when it all became so hilarious and exciting, I
> knew what I had done; inside all of us—so kind and thought-
> ful to everyone else—is a narcissist, an egotist, dying to
> get out!
>
> [Later] Helga is so funny—every time we meet she says,
> "Tell me again how we're going to act when we're skinny!"
> Whenever she asks, I do it; I dance around and shout, "We'll

tell everybody to go screw themselves! We'll look in the mirror three hours a day and never have time to clean or cook! We'll go bankrupt buying clothes! We will never feel guilty about anything! We will do whatever we damn please!" By this time she's falling on the floor, laughing. *'Don't, don't!'* she shrieks. "I'm laughing so hard I'll wet my pants!" and off she runs to her room, like a naughty child who has just gotten away with something.

That declaration of independence in the motel lobby never came to pass. I spend more time buying clothes and thinking about my appearance now, but clothes have not become an obsession—just an added dimension of pleasure. I still take care of a lot of people and work very hard. Eleanor Roosevelt remains my "ego ideal."

We are also people who are frightened of our anger. Fat is a shield that we think, in some primitive and childlike way, will keep our feelings inside—not let others know what we are really thinking and feeling. Children are terrified of losing control—they are afraid that *feeling* angry will make them *do* something terrible. Children who have temper tantrums are actually scared to death of what they are doing; they have lost control and their anger is spilling all over the place. Few of us who have been fat since childhood were tantrum-prone types. If we were angry at other people's expectations and demands, we drowned such feelings in an extra helping of chocolate pudding or mashed potatoes. And sometimes this pattern never seems to end. I wrote in my Durham journal:

> Kay arrived about a week ago. I like her at the same time that I could kill her! She's in her mid sixties, very straight-laced and proper. She has gained over two hundred pounds since she got married.
>
> She and her husband live in Washington. He comes from a wealthy and powerful family and she tells us jokingly about how he plucked her out of a symphony orchestra

where she was a violinist. "I was ten years younger than Ralph," she told us, "and he was exceedingly handsome and persuasive. I guess he had always gotten whatever he wanted, and it never crossed his mind that I could turn him down! He thought my music was a charming and admirable hobby and encouraged me to play for him—whenever I wasn't too busy having and raising the children."

She reads us parts of letters from her husband and children, who feel that losing weight is all just a matter of will power. One letter from her husband almost sent me through the ceiling, but somehow I managed to keep my mouth shut! He wrote, "You could just as well diet at home and take care of your responsibilities. If you just didn't eat anything for a year, you could still be living off your fat."

What drives me wild is how *sweet* she is.

She giggles when it would be appropriate to scream! And yet, like so many of us, she is expressing anger in an indirect way. How better to punish her husband for seducing her into giving up her music than to disgrace and shame him!

Before we are ready to diet, we need to give up the child's fantasy that anger can only create havoc. It is possible to express anger directly and appropriately; when we realize that, the number of trips to the refrigerator may diminish dramatically!

The terror of the unreal seems most often to come from childhood; the terror of the real is very much a part of the "here and now." I wrote in my Durham journal:

It's beginning to dawn on me that not everyone longs to go home, as I do. Quite a few of my fellow inmates are having more fun here than they ever have at home. They'd be crazy not to cheat—thereby prolonging the legitimacy of their stay here! Some talk quite openly about how marvelous it is not to have to take care of anybody else. Edith is usually the catalyst who gets us going. The other day she came and sat down at our table and said very mysteriously, "I hear a strange and wonderful humming in my ears today." As soon as she had our complete attention, she added, "It is the glorious sound of my washing machine, turned on by my husband or the kids instead of me!"

I'm becoming more aware of how many people are beginning to face how unhappy they have been in the past. Sylvia says it straight out: "A lot of us avoided coming to a place like this and losing weight for as long as we possibly could. We don't want to face what we know we are going to have to do—change our lives or gain all the weight back."

Estelle gets terrible attacks of colitis. She says, "If I get thin, I will have to deal with the way my husband has treated me—like a piece of dirt. As long as I was fat, I figured I deserved to be married to the son of a bitch; if I get thin, I'll have to figure out if I want to go on putting up with it—or whether he might change. Anyway, every pound I lose brings the reality closer. I'm seeing a shrink here, and he says the colitis is a substitute for the weight. There must be a better way out of all this!"

The compulsion to eat is not only a response to the need to relieve tension, anxiety, unhappiness, loneliness, shyness—the frustrations of life. Beyond all that, it is a way to avoid finding out who we really are and who we need to be.

All the apparently separate terrors are really one big terror—the terror of being oneself. We who have been obese since we were children have been burying a deep, dark secret under all those layers of fat, and the secret is that we gave up the struggle to discover who we really are, who we needed to be—we gave up our own special songs to sing—for the love and approval of other people. A great many other adults do the same. A great many of them are not fat—they have other forms of self-punishment. Why did we choose food and being fat? Answering that question is the real detective work, and it takes us back to the very beginning of our lives.

2

It Almost Always Starts
in Childhood

Some years ago, a psychotherapist who was trying to help me explore my early recollections of being a fat child suggested I try to recall some actual experience and write it as a story. The following was the result:

> They had been making fun of her; they called her "fatty" and they laughed, because she fell down while trying to skate. There were three tall boys and the two prettiest girls in the fifth-grade class. Walking home from school, miserable, full of shame, she stopped in the candy store where they sold the "Italian Cremes." One cent each; dark, bitter chocolate with soft, creamy, sweet white centers. She bought ten of them that day and ate three as she walked to the apartment where she lived. She wondered where she would hide the rest so her mother wouldn't find them. But when she got home her mother kissed her, and smelled the candy. She said, "You aren't helping yourself at all—you could be such a pretty girl if only you'd make a little effort. You know the doctor says it will get harder and harder if you don't do it now." The child couldn't answer. More misery, more shame; and even more, a hopelessness—because all she could think of as she walked to her room and

shut the door was where she could hide the candy until bedtime, and what she could steal from the kitchen before suppertime.

When I wrote that, I was beginning to understand that child— but I hated her. Now I feel a great tenderness toward her, because I worked hard for a long time to understand where she came from.

The Hungry Baby

Shortly after writing that description of myself, I found myself caught in a pattern of compulsive eating that was the worst such episode I could recall. I was heartsick, terrified; by that time I had already been trying for many years to control my eating and to lose weight.

The therapist commented, "Maybe these are the death throes of your compulsion. Often when you are almost ready to give up a neurotic symptom, there is an unconscious panic. After all, you needed the behavior or it wouldn't have developed in the first place."

That night I had a dream. I was sitting alone at a small table in a tremendous room. I was very small and the vastness of the room was frightening. There was an overwhelming feeling of isolation and loneliness. Whereas most of my dreams tend to be active, this one was quiet—it had a feeling of emptiness and profound sadness. The little girl was not crying; she seemed suspended in a pain beyond crying.

I had no idea what the dream meant, but its mood enveloped me until my next therapy session. The therapist suggested that sometimes, when the person is so small and the room so vast, the dream can be a real memory of a real time. Did I have any idea where the room might be? I knew instantly; it was the dining room of the house I lived in during the first three

years of my life—a small private house in the Bronx. Now I
remembered that the dining room was actually not large at all
and that it was right next to the kitchen. Why had I felt that
it was such a vast hall? Because that's the way small children
see their environment. Most of us have had the experience of
going back to a street or a house where we lived as children
and exclaiming over how much smaller everything seems. But
why the sense of loneliness? I couldn't seem to deal with that
at all, and the more the therapist pressed me to answer that
question, the more I seemed to maneuver our conversation to
other issues.

The therapy session was almost over. I was going away for
ten days, and I was frightened. I knew something important
was happening and that I was leaving it unfinished. Then, as
I was putting on my coat, I began to sob. "Oh, my God," I
cried. "She told me, 'If you don't eat your lunch I can't stay
with you.'" Suddenly I was two or three years old. I could
not stop crying—I felt so lonely, so frightened.

It seemed so ridiculous to be making such a fuss. It was a
perfectly normal, ordinary experience—shared by most other
children, I'm sure. My mother had been sitting with me while
I ate my lunch—perhaps reading me a story. I must have become
too full or perhaps didn't like what I was eating, so she had
left me and gone into the kitchen; I was punished by her withdrawal because I wasn't eating.

The floodgates of memory and emotion opened. It wasn't that
one episode in the dining room, of course. By that time my
mother and I already had a long history of a disturbed relationship over food. From the moment I was born, food was fraught
with special emotions, special problems.

I was born in June of 1922, during a terrific heat wave. My
mother and I struggled valiantly to establish nursing, but apparently we both failed. I lost weight during the first few weeks
of my life. My mother was frantic with worry; I was starving.

My mother and I were caught in a psychological bind. My grandmother had died when my mother was four years old, and she had never fully recovered from that trauma. I'm sure she was anxious and tense about mothering. To fail at feeding me must have been a terrible blow. I was screaming to be fed and she couldn't feed me. In those days doctors preferred to postpone giving cow's milk until cooler weather. I suppose the milk wasn't pasteurized then, and it was kept in iceboxes. When I was finally put on cow's milk, my hunger was insatiable.

After the dream about the dining room, I began to regress to feelings I'd had as a tiny baby. I began to remember how I'd felt, long before I had had language—or thought in language. All I knew as I sat in the therapist's office was that I was shaken by feelings of terror, of a sense that I was in a life-and-death struggle for survival. *I was fighting for my life.*

Once we begin to have conscious memories of childhood, we can probe the ways in which food had subtle emotional meanings for us. What is far more difficult is to recall infantile memories of the time in our lives when there was no language. During the period when I began to reexperience preverbal feelings, it was as if a black abyss of nothingness whirred around me and inside me. There was a sense of wordless, primeval terror and at the same time of rage. All I could feel was a timelessness and a spacelessness; I was nowhere and everywhere; I was suspended endlessly—forever. For a few minutes I just hung there, unable to speak; when finally I began to try to verbalize it, all I could say was, "I was dying and there was nothing I could do to help myself. There was no time and no space—I was endlessly to starve."

Being able to recall these feelings was helpful to me on many levels—and I have written elsewhere (in *In Search of Myself and Other Children*) about the ways in which it helped me to understand infancy and early childhood in general. What I think I also understand now is that anytime a baby is hungry and alone, it must feel as if its suffering will go on forever. A baby can't think: Hey, calm down, kid—Ma's just in the next room and she's taking a little long to get her bathrobe on and heat up that bottle because she's half asleep." For the infant, without language, without perception of time and space, any discomfort or fear has to be magnified a thousand times.

While all infants must experience some such moments, those of us who became fat probably had other experiences that reinforced these early feelings of panic. But if you grow up in a household where food is not used as a way of pleasing or displeasing parents, if you are naturally a skinny baby who grows into a skinny kid, you are less likely to become a compulsive eater.

Food and Love

When I was a child, enlightened parents were under the influence of the first wave of behavioristic psychology. I still have some of the books my mother referred to for guidance—chief among them, a book by the father of behaviorism, John B. Watson. My mother was one of the earliest pioneers in the new field of child study. She was eager to approach parenthood in the ways recommended by the experts of that time. So, like many other children, I became a victim of the theories that were popular in the time into which I was born. I became rigidly fixed on my digestive system! At mealtimes I had to eat my vegetables first, then I got my meat and finally my dessert. I was toilet trained very early, and there was a rigid schedule for bowel movements—if you missed a day at the right hour, you got a dose of "syrup of figs" or an enema.

My mother was tense and overanxious about taking care of me, and some of the inflexibility was her own. I recall an episode when I was about five or six and was given scrambled eggs for breakfast. I didn't eat them. My mother said if I didn't eat them, I'd get them again for lunch. At lunchtime, they were cold and awful, and I refused them again. I got them once more for supper—and by then, with a good deal of gagging, I ate them. I'd lost that round. Eating had by then become the battle-ground in a struggle for power.

It seems clear that by the time I was three or four years old, food had become a comfort, a weapon, a currency for the ex-changing of emotions—love, anger, rebellion, passivity, acquies-cence, rejection. I was a good girl when I ate and a bad girl when I did not. If I didn't eat what was on my plate, my mother would leave me alone; and I suppose the depth of my anguish at that dining room table in the dream indicates that this experi-ence was somehow a recapitulation of the way I felt as a tiny infant—that I was all alone in the world, starving, struggling to survive.

When I was about three years old, we moved into the top floor of the brownstone where my grandparents lived. My grand-father had remarried and it was like moving into the best restau-rant in the city of Prague! My grandmother was a gourmet Czechoslovakian chef and my grandfather her devoted and en-thusiastic audience. I remember more about food during the next few years in that house than about almost anything else. I remember waiting every day for my grandfather to come home from work, and the game we played of my trying to find out which pocket had the candy he'd bought me. And I remember my Aunt Edith or Uncle Edward taking me to the penny candy store on the corner. But most of all, I remember "Ottie"—Ottilie, my grandmother—letting me help her stretch the strudel dough on the dining room table, or blanch the almonds for prune yeast cakes, or lick the whipped cream bowl when she made a chocolate roll cake. Being on the kitchen staff was the happiest job I've ever had!

A few years later, eating became being a bad girl. People were beginning to worry; I was getting too heavy. While I might have experienced anger and withdrawal of love before because

I wouldn't eat, now I was getting disapproving looks because I could pack away as much as my grandfather. Food, the Great Comforter, had become off limits.

My mother died in 1973. Despite the problems we shared, we had had a profoundly loving relationship; the more I came to understand the influences and experiences that had shaped her life, the more I felt compassion and love for her. When she died, my grief was intense. A few months after her death, I began eating compulsively again, after quite a long period in which I'd eaten sensibly and lost weight slowly. Suddenly I was again stuffing myself with sweets. One night, after this had been going on for some time, I had a sequence of frightening dreams. I woke up terribly upset at four in the morning and burst into tears. My husband awoke, and we began to talk. (There are tremendous advantages to being married to a psychologist!) It soon became clear that all the dreams had one theme: in some primitive and childlike way, my unconscious had been telling me I could get my mother back, if only I would eat. Quietly, Larry said, "It's terribly sad, but you must face the fact that *she has not gone into the kitchen this time.*" Food and love had become twisted and entangled to such a degree that even though I was now fifty, the child in me was screaming for my mother, trying to bring her back from the dead by being a good little girl—and eating.

The First Self-Image

It is hard for us to believe that we are still the victims of the fantasies and irrationalities of childhood, but I am sure this is the case. One evening in Durham, four or five of us were agreeing that we often begin to feel sick when we lose weight. I wrote in my journal:

> Billy told us, "The doctors kept telling me that being fat would kill me, but I kept feeling as if I would die if I didn't

eat." Judy told us, "As soon as I start dieting, I begin to have crazy fears that I'll disappear." Ben said, "When I start dieting, I get all kinds of aches and pains which no doctor is able to explain." I think we all react to early experiences we can't even remember.

David, twenty-one years old, weighed 340 pounds when he came to Durham. He would stick to his diet for a few days and then go on a gigantic binge. We became friends after a while and I wrote about him in my journal:

> I met David in the lobby, where I was waiting for the limousine to take me to the airport for my first "furlough" home. I told him I was scared to death; could I go on dieting in my normal environment? I told him how I felt as a child, hoping he would begin to reminisce with me. But he didn't—he just listened. When the limousine came, he carried my bag outside. "Thanks, Eda," he said. "Don't worry about me. By the time I was seven years old, in second grade, I weighed 115 pounds. The other kids started calling me 'that fat boy,' and that's how I have thought of myself every minute since then."

Whether we have become fat children mostly because of hereditary tendencies, or because we were born big, or because we were underfed or overfed, by the time we are six or seven the image we have of ourselves begins to interfere with our capacity to deny ourselves the comfort of food. Almost any child who is told by adults that he must lose weight is likely to assume that this means he is abnormal—not like everyone else. Children don't have the capacity for refined judgments. One is either fat or thin, beautiful or ugly, smart or dumb.

One area of insecurity is likely to lead to many. By second grade I also felt dumb; it seemed quite natural to be fat *and* dumb.

I also dreaded gym classes, where I felt clumsy and inept. I remember one particular episode of torment in sixth grade. As part of our arithmetic lessons, the teacher brought in a scale to weigh and measure all of us, in order to teach the meaning of "average"—taking the total and then dividing by the number in the class. The weighing was done and recorded in front of everyone. I weighed more than anyone except for one very tall boy. The teacher explained how the thin and tiny and the tall and fat students influenced the average. It was hell, pure and simple.

In junior and senior high school there were also "public weighings," done by the school nurse. One nurse tried to shame me by shouting out the bad news—"to *make* you go on a diet!" she said self-righteously. One nurse was kind—she whispered the dread information to whoever was recording the statistics—but everyone knew why she was whispering.

When you are young and in deadly competition with all your peers, anything that represents a feeling of being handicapped in some way spreads into every other area of your life.

Fat children tend to use the fact of being overweight as an explanation for the perfectly normal doubts and misgivings of childhood. I never met a child who didn't sometimes feel shy, dumb, ugly or unpopular. Thin kids blame their troubles on having freckles, or poor coordination, or curly hair, or straight hair, or being nearsighted, or having a high voice, or a low voice, or being teacher's pet. Fat kids never have to look very far for explanations of insecurity; anything—everything—becomes related to being overweight, and all problems are dealt with through the momentary comfort and appeasement of eating.

The Punishments Fit Our Crimes

I wrote in my Durham journal:

> David told me that last night he ate two whole pizzas. He has gained back six pounds in the past few days. I told

him that I knew it was hard to get over hating oneself and then punishing oneself. He looked startled. I asked him what "terrible things" he had done when he was a little boy. In deadly seriousness, he began to think about how awful he had been. "When I was six years old, I stole a dollar from my father," he told me. He waited to see my reaction, and when I laughed, he added, with growing enthusiasm, "I used to pinch my sister when she was a baby—but not hard enough so it would show, and I would lie like hell about it. I hated my brother; I began to smoke when I was nine; I once started a fire in the basement, and I lied to my mother about going to a movie instead of a Boy Scout meeting." I told him, "Listen, dummy, I majored in *child psychology*—and I am here to tell you that all of those 'crimes' were the normal behavior of a nice kid." David looked at me and said, "If I wasn't so bad, why did my father punish me all the time?"

Too few parents realize what punishment really means to many children. It is not a deterrent to further "bad" behavior, but rather confirms for the child that he is a bad person. We think we punish children for their shortcomings, and we hope the punishment will improve their behavior. Unfortunately, what usually happens is that the punishment simply relieves the child of the heavy burden of guilt he already feels. Children assume that when they misbehave it is because they are terrible people and therefore they deserve to be punished. They do not understand that they are merely behaving childishly because they are children. There is a vast difference between saying to a child, "I am going to punish you for being so bad and stealing from me," and saying something like, "I'm going to punish you for taking that money because I have to try to help you remember that you must not take things that belong to other people. All children do this sometimes and grownups have to help them learn to stop doing it."

Rarely do adults explain the difference to children between

being childish because you are a child, and being "bad." This seems a simple, perhaps even an innocuous point. It is my belief, though, after studying children for most of my life, that it is the root of most feelings of self-hatred.

Adolescence

Adolescence is the time when self-hatred reaches monumental proportions. Everyone, including the most beautiful and handsome, the athletes and the geniuses, feels insecure and uncertain. Adolescence is a time for natural rebellion against parental authority; it is also the time for the normal emergence of powerful sexual feelings, and both parents and children tend to become too anxious, too threatened, to communicate with each other effectively.

When I was about eleven years old I got rheumatic fever, which at that time was treated mostly by total bed rest. I went to bed chubby and got up some months later, awkward, overweight and self-conscious. My classmates had been moving right along; they were going to dancing school and a few sophisticates had even started dating. From then on, my mother's exhortations about losing weight came almost daily. She wrote me long letters (even though we lived in the same house) about "will power" and "self-control" and "how pretty you *could* be." If I didn't lose weight I would ruin my future life. I knew my mother loved me, and I was sure she was right. It was because of my depravity that I could not stop eating. What I did not understand until many years later was that her feelings about herself, her own insecurity, were partly responsible for what was happening between us. What she could not see was how much I was suffering, without her exhortations, pleadings, warnings. I felt ugly and clumsy; I hated team sports and went through the hinges of hell when teams were being formed, mortified that I might be chosen last. Looking back now, I have a different perspective on those years. I had many close friends. I was well liked by my teachers. I was editor of the literary magazine, and was even nominated for president of the student council. Not exactly a tragic life! But I *felt* as if being overweight was the most important thing about me.

Everyone I met at Durham who had been fat as a child seemed to have had similar experiences. During adolescence, the neurotic interaction between parent and child about being overweight becomes even more intense. Mother is anxious and frightened; is her child going to be as unattractive as perhaps the mother feels *she* is? She is sure she has failed and her guilt is profound. The more guilty she feels, the more she nags. The child (and this seems true for both boys and girls) feels ugly and ashamed. Eating increasingly becomes a way of comforting oneself—and also of punishing the parent, who is finally vulnerable. When I was little, I ate what my mother told me to eat; as a teen-ager, I learned that I could control her by eating what she didn't want me to eat. Since most adolescents need to find some area of rebellion against parents—and we who are fat are usually children who do not rebel too easily—food becomes the weapon we are most comfortable with.

In Durham, I noticed a very marked difference between the older and younger patients. The majority of the middle-aged seemed reasonably well adjusted; they were neurotic on the subject of food, but then everybody is neurotic about something! The kids, on the other hand—the teen-agers and young adults— tended often to be seriously disturbed. Some were sullen and defiant; many smoked and drank heavily, and were experimenting with hard drugs. My impression was that they *all* cheated. It seemed to me that most of them thought: I am here because my parents didn't know what else to do with me. They felt more ostracized by the thin culture than the older people did.

At least, in middle age, fat is tolerated; among the young there is real discrimination and rejection. A great many of the young patients seemed to be acting out against parental rejection and authority. It was my opinion that they should *not* have been on a diet program that did not include psychological counseling and adult supervision, which they needed desperately.

It seems to me that adolescence is the most difficult time for a child to diet: the feelings of worthlessness are so pronounced, there is such inner turmoil and confusion, and the need to rebel is so strong. For many adolescents, the emergence of sexual drives becomes a source of panic, and they use food as a way of hiding, repressing their feelings. Eating a large plate of mashed potatoes or a whole blueberry pie becomes a way of burying sexual urges. And if no amount of overstuffing can sub-due those disturbing feelings, that thickening layer of fat will help to keep others away—and protect one from temptation. Many fat people sense unconsciously that they have a passionate and sensual nature. The adolescent may be too fearful to deal with such feelings: There are and always have been teen-agers who have been afraid of their emerging sexuality. Some get migraine headaches, some get religion; some even have nervous breakdowns. But if fat has become a familiar escape route, it tends to be the evasion of choice. It was most assuredly mine.

Fathers

Ever since Freud observed that what we become is related to our childhood experiences, mothers have really been getting it in the neck! It seems very unfair to me. I tried a number of times while in Durham to find people who felt that their fathers had played a major part in their weight problems, but no one was ready to admit such a possibility.

Even if our fathers did nag or make fun of us, or ignore the problem, or entice us to eat—giving us the same double messages we got from our mothers—our most intense struggles were with our mothers. (Of course, it's a comparatively recent development for fathers to share an active role in the raising of children.) There was, however, one interesting exception in Durham, which I described in my journal:

> Carole's father has come to visit two or three times, and each time, while ranting and railing that Carole isn't doing well enough to warrant her staying here, he has also sabotaged her dieting by enticing her to eat out at the best restaurants in the area. I think he wants her to stay fat to keep boys away so that Carole will continue to be his "Dollbaby." However, I think Carole is very determined to free herself and become more independent.

As fathers become more actively engaged in all aspects of child raising, this emphasis on the mother as the creator of attitudes about eating will undoubtedly lessen. What seems to have happened frequently up to now is that fathers have tended to reinforce maternal behavior more by omission than commission; they just don't get involved. Or they may reinforce what is already happening by attitudes that seem more benign and passive but that may actually be as influential as anything mother is doing or saying.

I cannot recall that my father ever nagged me about eating too much. He, too, came from a large family, in which cooking and eating were emphasized, fat children were considered healthier than skinny ones, and sharing food was an essential part of communicating love. He also seemed to me to be far more concerned with my brain than with my body. I remember that in high school I had a friend who always complained bitterly because her father insisted on going shopping with her and had final approval of anything she bought. This made her furious—

but I was jealous because it seemed wonderful to me that her father cared so much about the way she looked. While I was in Durham, something happened that reminded me of one particular episode of my adolescence:

> Kay has lost twenty pounds. Yesterday she went to a very fancy shop here and bought a new dress, two sizes smaller than the ones she's been wearing, because her husband and daughter were coming to visit for the weekend and she wanted to surprise them. I was in the lobby when they arrived. Kay was all dressed up and very excited. Neither one of them said *one word* about how great she looked, or congratulated her on her weight loss. Her husband complained about the plane being late and her daughter said the food on the plane was so awful she couldn't eat it—so where could they go to get some lunch? Kay's eyes just went dead. Suddenly I remembered having had what I imagine must have been the same feeling when I was sixteen and going to my first formal party on New Year's Eve. I remember every detail of the dress I wore—turquoise chiffon, draped and cut in a Grecian style. I thought it was the most perfect dress I'd ever seen, and when I was all dressed, I felt beautiful. My parents were getting ready to go out too, and I remember that I was longing for my father to notice my new dress, but he said nothing.
>
> A few minutes later my uncle and aunt arrived to pick up my parents. Uncle Henry took one look at me and boomed, "Look at this gorgeous creature!" He hugged me and made me turn around several times, and kept exclaiming about what a beautiful woman I was becoming. Suddenly I felt so sad because my father hadn't been the one who said it.

Having a father who was kind and loving, but who seemed disinterested in my feelings about becoming a woman, reinforced my feelings of self-disgust. Passivity or seeming indifference can play as important a role as too much pressure.

Rebellion and Guilt

Recently my aunt and I were comparing notes about growing up in households where food was an important way of communicating feelings. She was a skinny child, has never been overweight a day of her life and never overeats. Also, she hates desserts! "Why is it," she asked me, "that you start salivating the minute you hear the words 'cocoa cake' or 'almond crescents' and I couldn't care less? If getting fat is psychological, we should be the same!" But we are *not* the same because she had a different mother, who was not anxious about food; she nursed successfully; she has a thin body build; and for her eating never became mixed with other issues.

Childhood obesity is a combination of predisposition and environment. In order for a pattern of overeating to become fixed and unchanging, parents must be giving mixed messages: I'll love you if you eat; if you don't eat you'll get sick; I want you to be strong. Now it is time to stop eating; eating will make you ugly and unpopular. Food is wonderful; food is terrible. I give you food because I love you. I take food away from you because I love you.

One of the problems in trying to lose weight is that many of us feel we are doing something that our parents unconsciously probably don't want us to do and that makes us feel guilty. They *say* that they are worried about our being fat and they try to make us diet, but unconsciously our being fat makes for a kind of dependency that some parents don't want to give up. As long as we remain fat, we are still their little children. If we begin to lose weight, this becomes a symbol of rebellion: our getting thin scares parents in much the same way it might scare a spouse, or even one's own children. The way it scares *us!* We are, after all, fighting *for our own lives.* The people around us who have become very dependent on us see this as a declaration of independence: we may escape from their demands on us. We gain back the weight as an act of compliance; we are too nice to hurt other people's feelings.

Helping Fat Children

Spring arrived while I was in Durham. By the beginning of March, the forsythia was blooming, and the crocuses and daffodils. As I began to perceive myself as no longer fat, I exulted in the world of nature. I saw five cardinals and heard my very first mockingbird. One day, listening to the sounds of birds singing, I found myself in tears. I was missing my mother. I wanted to tell her what had happened to me. There is no one who wanted this for me more than she did—no one who loved me more or cared more deeply. *I wanted her to see me now!* I wanted to tell her that I knew how much she wanted to help me, and that her failure was the fault of her own childhood anguish and the times in which she and I lived together, when there was so little understanding of the misery experienced by the fat child. I wanted to tell her that maybe, out of the pain of our experience, other children might be helped.

On the basis of my own life experience and everything I have learned from others, it seems to me that there are three basic principles involved in dealing with childhood obesity: one must (1) avoid repeating one's own past history; (2) refuse to allow eating to become loaded with extraneous and complex emotions; and (3) acknowledge that it is the *child's* problem and allow him or her the necessary autonomy to deal with it.

The fact that my daughter never became a fat person is a miracle of good fortune, owed to a set of genes and chromosomes which defied overeating, and to my constant awareness of that first basic principle, *not* to repeat the patterns of my childhood. I struggled constantly because my natural tendency was to be rigid about food, to be inflexible about rules, and to use food as a way of communicating love. I failed much of the time, but I knew that I had made the grade and become more relaxed about food than my mother when Wendy arrived home after spending a weekend at a friend's house and said, as she ate her breakfast the next morning, "It's great to be back to *normal!* All you get at Jane's house for breakfast is eggs or cereal." At the moment, she was eating a hamburger. I felt as if I'd been given the Mother of the Year Award for flexibility!

Whenever our children have problems we begin to feel guilty, and the more guilty we feel about our children's shortcomings, the more we gravitate to old ways of handling anxiety—and in our case that means using the giving and taking away of food as a substitute for dealing directly with problems.

If we become fat, chances are we have become accustomed to junk foods. We are constantly enticed to buy frozen dinners, potato chips, Devil Dogs, cheeseburgers, french fries, and thirty-one flavors of ice cream. We are bombarded by television advertising, and by those endless and proliferating food chains that cover every road we drive on, emitting smells that start our salivary glands going.

There is no way to protect our children from obesity, high blood pressure, diabetes and a gloomy assortment of other diseases, except to make up our minds not to have any junk in the house. An occasional spree—because we are human—is unavoidable and necessary. Five poisonous hot dogs at a baseball game, three candy apples at the circus, two Hershey bars in a movie, aren't exactly healthy, but fun is fun, and it won't kill us to indulge ourselves occasionally. What we need to do, though, is to develop habits of shopping and eating that will tend to become unconscious behavior after we practice for a while. We need to become more creative about how and what we cook. We need to have lots of healthy snacks around the house that give pleasure and don't make children feel deprived—raisins, figs, dates, bananas, nuts, and all those new and enticing goodies we are beginning to find in health food stores.

I think it is a cop-out for parents to fuss about the terrible ads on television for candy, and cereals made of sugar, and other harmful ingredients. If enough families would stop buying this junk, the companies would go out of business in a week, and the networks would have to find something else to sell. The buck stops *in front of* the television set.

As an adult, I had to find other ways of giving myself pleasure than through food. We can do the same thing for overweight children. Depending on a child's interests, there are many ways of feeding a soul. Going on a camping trip, visiting Disneyland (carrying a bag of fruits and nuts!), reading an extra story together, going to a movie or a concert, taking guitar lessons, buying some new clothes, are all helpful kinds of things to do if it is understood that such extra luxuries or pleasures are intended to help a child solve a problem, not as rewards for good behavior.

If we are fat, we are likely to prefer sitting to standing and lying down to sitting! One of the most important ways that parents can help overweight children is to *stop using the family car*. That's good for the budget and air pollution and the energy crisis—but most of all it's a good way to help people start moving again. Walking is a skill we are rediscovering. Bicycles are a perfectly adequate means of getting just about anywhere a child needs to go. The whole family can jog together, play tennis, swim—do anything except spend most of their time sitting in a car or in front of a television set.

Then there is that factor present in most of our backgrounds— a natural feeling that wasting food is deplorable. For many families, memories of hunger go back just a generation or two and subtly influence their lives. While I was in Durham, we often compared notes about this:

> Today a group of us were comparing notes about what nationality it was that was starving when we were children

and for whom we had to finish the food on our plates. When I was a child it was the "starving Armenians." Susie (22) says it was Africans in general and Biafrans in particular. We each had some country for which we were shamed into eating more food than we wanted or needed. I told them the story of how shocked Larry and I were when our daughter broke the bind of generations by looking us square in the eye and saying, "How will it help the Korean children if I eat this?" We *can* interrupt this seemingly inevitable pattern, but it takes hard work and constant self-awareness.

Getting to the second principle, if we have learned anything from our own life experiences, it is surely that food can become inextricably confused with other emotional issues. Parents often get very frightened if they don't feel love for their children all the time, and they offer food to assuage the resulting guilt. But nobody can love a child every single minute. Anger, ambivalence, jealousy, exhaustion—even dislike—are perfectly normal human feelings and nothing to be ashamed of. Such feelings only lead to disaster when parents try to keep them buried. It is far better to admit honestly, "You're making me so mad I can't see straight!" than to offer a child five more cookies or a pint of ice cream and hope he or she won't know how we are really feeling.

By sensitizing ourselves to the fact that we learned early and well to accept food as a substitute for honest communication and unconditional love, we can begin to control such behavior successfully. Children do not have to be loved every minute. If we can tolerate human imperfection, they will be able to as well. It will do them more good to observe our ambivalences than to have food stuffed into their mouths while we do a slow internal burn. It is not necessary to behave in loving ways all the time—but there is a slight complication: children *do* need unconditional loving in order to grow well.

What I mean is this: Children can tolerate the broad range of honest human emotions, expressed in the course of their daily lives—and if it doesn't throw us, it won't throw them. But what they need in addition—like a quiet river flowing steadily beneath the surface of living experiences—is the feeling that they are perceived as wonderful just as they are; that they need not do anything to deserve or earn love; that we do not love them because they are smart, pretty, handsome, cute, sweet, talented, or the right size and shape. I began to understand this in a new way after I had lost fifty pounds. I wrote in my journal:

> It is so interesting to see how different people react when they see me. The ones who make me feel wonderful are the ones who are pleased that *I* am so happy, but who say that I have only "revealed" what they already knew about me. Barbara said, "I'm so glad if you are over your miseries— but to me you were always beautiful." Maria said, "Since only the essential you has ever mattered to me, I shall not miss the superfluous you!" Peggy wrote, "It is good to contemplate you minus agony," and when I asked Wendy if she was nervous about seeing me, she said, "I'll be seeing the real you—the person I've always known was there." I keep thinking about what my mother would say. I know she would care more than anyone else, but I suspect she would say the wrong thing—something like, "You see? I always *told* you you could be pretty." Or "Now you can understand why I nagged you so much." As a child I interpreted this kind of language as representing conditional love; all things were possible *if only* I had will power. What reinforces my current struggle is that nobody who loves me really cared one way or the other except that *they didn't want me to suffer.* What a simple idea that is—and yet so difficult a message for parents to communicate to children!

Children need to know that they are lovable in their very essence—with no conditions, no claims. They also need to feel that the people who love them want to do everything they can to help them, but that it is up to the child to want to change for his or her own sake, and not to please anyone else.

It is terribly easy to fall into the pattern of unconsciously encouraging children to eat more than they need to for healthy growing. One characteristic of those of us who were fat children is that we tried so hard to please our parents and were seldom openly rebellious. It certainly made life easier for our parents to live with a child who was obsequious rather than rebellious. It is much harder to raise kids who fight back, who struggle to be themselves and to satisfy their needs rather than their parents'. At one extreme is the outwardly placid child who is really feeling angry and frustrated at too many controls, who drowns his or her feelings in a quart of pistachio ice cream; and at the other extreme is the child who openly defies parental controls, and prefers to be a little devil than to pacify himself with a devil's food cake!

Parents like to be loved too! We enjoy it when our children are happy. And food is such an easy way to make a person of any age feel happy! How can we turn down a request for just one more piece of birthday cake? How could anyone not offer a child a bowl to lick?

What I think is most helpful is facing the fact that food is a universal source of pleasure. We and our children need to break the rules once in a while and splurge; that's all right, if we avoid hidden messages and don't play emotional games with food, substituting it for the expression of feelings.

The final basic principle involves the understanding that when a child is overweight, it is his or her own problem. We know from our experience that nagging, pleading, warning, bribing or deprivation never helped us to solve the problem.

As I look back to years of anguish about being fat, it seems to me that my mother and I talked about it a lot but it was more a monologue than a dialogue; I could not tell her how *I* was feeling. If you have to face the problem of an obese child, try to offer help in whatever ways *your child* wants you to. Rather than telling the child how you feel, try to elicit how he or she feels. Ask questions instead of making statements. If you think it would be helpful to talk about how you felt as a child, do so—but not to such an extent as to cut off your child's expression of his or her own experience. Suggest that you talk about it as two friends, not as enemies in a struggle for power and control. Try to indicate that you share a common human problem, and don't focus attention on the success or failure of dieting until the child asks for such help.

Once your child is able to talk about his or her feelings, is able to say, "I'm miserable, I'm ashamed, I'm hopeless, I'm angry—it isn't fair," then it is possible to become an ally, to say, "What can I do to help you?"

Food ought never to be used as a punishment or a reward. When a child begins eating compulsively, we need to ask ourselves: Is this to escape our demands and expectations? Is this child really angry at us? Does he need to tell us about some negative feelings, in order to clear the air and let us know where and how we may be expecting too much, setting impossible goals or imposing too many limits? We need to be clear with kids that eating is no substitute for solving relationship problems—that we prefer confrontation to gluttony. It's harder to listen to a child tell you how angry he is, but we of all people should know that's a small price to pay for helping a child meet life directly, rather than through the bland mist of a marshmallow sundae.

One of the things that now seem most important to me is the child's right to her own failures. A twelve-year-old girl asks her parents to help her lose ten pounds; she works out a diet, she discusses it with the doctor, she does some of the special shopping and cooking. Wonderful—she's developing some autonomy in working out her problem. Then one day she feels lousy because her best friend has deserted her; she has two egg creams after school, and feeling even worse, takes a Sara Lee cake out of the freezer at home and eats the whole thing before supper. If she feels she has failed and will be a great disappointment to her parents, she is likely to keep this fall from grace to herself. But if she and her family have anticipated just this kind of eventuality, it is more likely to be taken in stride; tomorrow is another day, to begin again.

Failure is a built-in factor in all life experiences, irrespective of will power or motivation. I try now to imagine what might have happened if I had felt free to admit it the day I ate all those Italian Cremes—and if I could have explained why. Suppose my mother had hugged me sympathetically and said, "*Of course* you'll fail sometimes—you're only human, you know. But you are succeeding more days than you are failing, and that must give you a great deal of satisfaction." I know it wouldn't have hurt—and it might have helped a lot.

Looking back on my childhood and my parenting during my child's adolescence, I am convinced that parents sabotage growth even while they consciously say they want to see it occur. Perhaps it is partly the fear of the coming necessary separation. When a child grows up and moves away from us psychologically, we are, after all, losing part of ourselves. Maybe we don't allow ourselves the opportunity to mourn adequately for the lost child. The emerging adult can never be our baby again. It is the end of a deeply symbolic relationship.

The hardest thing in the world is to really allow a young person to test himself. For a young person to move toward adult decision making, there must come a time when parents no longer take responsibility for that decision making.

Inside each child is the capacity, the possibility, for courage, will power, self-direction. It cannot be elicited by the despairing sound of: "If only you would . . ." It *can* be encouraged and reinforced by: "I know how you feel and what a struggle it must be. You are special and wonderful and beautiful. Let me know if I can help you reveal yourself more fully." By the time

I was fifty-four, I was able to say that to myself. It is sad that I could not hear those words when I was young. But how happy I would be if some parent, reading this, could say it to his or her child.

3

Shock:
When Obesity
Starts with
a Trauma

While it is true that the majority of fat adults were also fat children, I discovered a great many exceptions during my months in Durham. People get fat for a lot of different reasons. I wrote in my journal:

> It's strange—the first two or three people I am getting to know here were never overweight until the last year or two. One is a tiny lady, Dee, who told me that she had gained fifty pounds during the first six months after her husband's death. She has already lost forty-five pounds here. I would guess she's about sixty years old. Then there's a younger woman, Jessie, who told me that in her entire adult life she never weighed over 125 pounds—until her six-year-old son fell into a building excavation and died. Now she weighs two hundred pounds.
>
> At first my reaction was one of great surprise; I had never

thought about the fact that some people get fat all of a
sudden, after something awful has happened to them. How
dumb of me! I've been so wrapped up in my own childhood
problems that I just never thought about obesity as a psycho-
somatic reaction to tragedy or adversity. If I believe that
people can get migraine headaches, rheumatoid arthritis,
ulcers, colitis—even cancer—because of lowered resistance
due to stress, why in the world should compulsive eating
not be a psychological response to shock?

What I learned as I talked with others was that grief and obesity
were frequently associated.

Normal Grief

I soon realized that at least a third of my fellow patients in
Durham had never been fat until they had experienced some
horrible shock or loss. Once I became aware of this, it seemed
a very natural reaction to anguish; food is the earliest and most
primitive comfort we experience in life, and regression is a natural response to great pain.

Eventually I found myself dividing the group into those who
used food as a way to assuage their natural feelings of grief
during a normal period of mourning, and those who became
neurotically bound to overeating. As the process of recovery
began, the first group became aware of the fact that they had
gained a great deal of weight and quickly set about losing it.
Dee and Jessie were in that group. They had suffered terribly,
but they described their mourning period as open and uninhib-
ited; they had expressed their feelings in ways that had eventually brought them comfort. Dee told me: "I come from a very
orthodox Jewish family; our religion gives us a way to express
how terrible we feel right away when we sit *shiva*, and when
everyone comes to see us, and we cry and hug each other a
lot. My husband and I had thirty-five wonderful years together.

Not that he was any saint—believe me, we had our troubles—but he was the right man for me and that makes me luckier than half the women I know. For a few months I was crazy; I couldn't sleep, so I ate. Suddenly I woke up one morning and I was *fat!* But I'm taking it off quickly and I realize that eating a lot of rich food comforted me. Now I don't need it anymore."

Jessie said: "At first I blamed myself for Richie's death: I was guilty, I had killed him. I began stuffing myself and taking tranquilizers and sleeping pills, to keep the agony under control. That was my first mistake. I have two other kids and I didn't want to let them see how much I was suffering. That was my second mistake. After a couple of months I realized I was getting fat and that my husband and kids had become strangers. I let them in on how I felt and of course they were suffering as much as I was. Three months after the funeral, we all cried together. Then I tried to deal with my guilt. There was no way I could have known that there was a hole that Richie could have crawled through. Then I began to be furious at Richie! That was crazy time; I was screaming at a child for daring to do this to me! Last month I decided it was time to pull myself together; life goes on."

I felt that both these women had experienced their grief in ways that were helping them to recover. They would doubtless be able to lose the weight they had gained and go on with their lives.

Depression: Excessive Grief and Mourning

But there was another group, in which obesity seemed to be a more serious and intense symptom of deep depression. Compulsive eating that cannot be controlled, even when it has led to very serious and dangerous complications (hypertension, diabetes, etc.), can be a manifestation of a mourner's repressed feelings of guilt and ambivalence about his or her loss. People who react in such a way tend to dislike bothering other people with their feelings; they are not screamers or groaners or complainers—they have always tried to internalize their pain. Because they are unable to "bother others" with normal feelings of rage and despair, their inner tension becomes so great that the resulting stress causes some combination of physical and psychological illness. I wrote in my Durham journal;

> Harry is such a sad person; he has isolated himself from the world. His wife died about three years ago. He doesn't want to see his son or grandchildren. He retired from his job and became a recluse. He began eating compulsively until he was obese. Then he had a heart attack and his doctor sent him here. He's lonely and depressed—still grieving. He's one of those people who cannot accept the fact that every relationship is ambivalent. He speaks of his wife as if she was perfect—"an angel." That's why he can't recover—he can't deal with the fact that it was a *human* relationship and that he didn't love her every single minute! Or that he is a whole human being, even without her presence. He's being very proper, very polite—and utterly miserable.

Harry stayed in Durham only a few weeks. He could not face his own humanity and so he kept on eating.

The Fear of Facing Oneself

The most courageous among us learn to use life's tragedies for growing, becoming more than we have been. I wrote in my journal;

> I am convinced that Helga will lose some weight while she is here—and then gain it all back as soon as she goes home. My first impression of her was the stereotype of a fat, jolly lady, but as I got to know her, the facade lifted and she seemed so tragic. For many years she and her hus-

band tried to have children but couldn't; then it was necessary for her to have a hysterectomy. After that they tried for a long time to adopt a child and lived through several gruesome disappointments. When they had pretty much given up hope, they were finally able to adopt a teen-age boy. They knew he had had terrible life experiences and had been a behavior problem, but Helga was certain that her tremendous need to mother a child would solve his problems.

For a year or two it looked as if it might work out; Helga devoted her life, all her energies, to rehabilitating this child. Then he was caught by the police as part of a gang involved in an armed robbery in which a man was killed. He is now in prison, without possibility of parole for twenty-five years. Helga gained one hundred pounds in the next two years. "I needed so much to be a mama," she says, weeping, "and look what I did." She is convinced that her guilt is as great as her child's, and there is no way to change her mind. I think that she takes this inflexible emotional stance because her anger at the child is more unbearable to face than anger at herself. The truth is, I think, that she is in a rage against this child who didn't appreciate what she was doing for him, and who didn't live up to her expectations.

The kind of trauma that plays directly into problems of personal identity is one that hits a person right in the middle of his very being: when what was lost was the major relationship of a lifetime—a place, a job, a person, even one's own goals in life—in which one has invested all of one's psychological energy. The sudden onset of compulsive eating has to do with the fact that whatever the tragic event may be, it has set in motion a whole process of reevaluating one's essential identity as a human being. Nothing is more likely to make us anxious than being forced to examine our own lives! Few things can create more stress. I met several people in Durham who seemed to be in this situation:

Lucy is twenty-three and weighs 210 pounds. She gained sixty pounds in one year! She told me, "I come from a small town in South Dakota—and for as long as I can remember, my whole life was focused on *getting out of there!* I was born smart, I guess, and school bored me, the church bored me, my family bored me. I had this terrific fantasy that I'd go away to college and then I'd go to New York and be very successful and sophisticated. I worked my way through a small college about one hundred miles from home. It was a terrific struggle but it didn't matter—I knew where I was going! I worked for a year after college, living at home, saving every penny, and then I went to New York to look for a job. I had all these ideas from the movies about how New York would look, all the fascinating people I'd meet—how I'd never be bored again. Well, I was right about one thing—I sure wasn't bored! But I was scared to death; I was lonely and shy; I was *homesick!*

"I had no idea how to go about getting a job or how to find a place to live or how to meet people. Everything frightened me. Instead of a glamorous apartment, all I could afford was a furnished room. The noise, the traffic, people rushing around, not knowing anybody—it sure wasn't living up to my fantasy. I began stuffing myself constantly—at work, over weekends. I would sit in my room telling myself I should go to a museum, but instead I'd go to a bakery, buy a lot of pastries, and sit in my room and eat. I got a job as a receptionist and one of the women in the office finally said something to me about how fat I was getting. She was very nice about it. She told me she had come here [to Durham] and she said I should take a leave of absence and come here. I borrowed some money from my family, and after I get back to my normal size, I'm going to go home for a while and think things over. I think I'll want to go back to New York, but this time I'll be dealing with reality, not a childhood fantasy!"

Sometime later, I met Janice:

> She's a lovely and gentle woman who seems to have been through hell. She was never overweight as a child or as a young adult, but it began to creep up on her through a miserable marriage, a disastrous divorce, and serious financial problems. And then, just as she was beginning to get on her feet, her only son began to have all kinds of problems—he married a girl who ultimately committed suicide, and then dumped his child on Janice's doorstep to raise. She adored this grandson, took care of him until, at the age of eight, he developed bone cancer and died. She is very overweight now, and has had two minor strokes. She was more dead than alive when she decided to hock everything and come here. She knows that she is going through an existential crisis—should she start all over again, or should she just give up and die? I told her it seemed to me she had already made the decision to live or she wouldn't have come here. She seemed relieved to hear that!

> [Later] I can see now why Janice began to try to kill herself. The one role that seems to have satisfied her has been mothering—first her son and then her grandson. There is something deliciously childlike about her—she must have been a marvelous companion for a child. It was the one aspect of her life in which she felt competent and happy. Her parents thought she was stupid, her husband was cruelly rejecting, she was never trained for any profession— but how she comes to life when she talks about being a mother and grandmother! And then to feel that somehow she had failed even there—to protect her children—must have been the ultimate blow to her very ragged and uncertain self-esteem. Today she told me that while she was gaining so much weight she could never talk about her pain to anyone. In fact, for a year after his death, she never mentioned her grandson's name. We sat in a beautiful little park today and she wept on and off for several hours—

something she says she has never done in front of another person before. It's high time!

Going on with Life

The loss of someone we love can serve to remind us of how precious the human experience is—and there can follow a kind of inner declaration that life must not be wasted. I saw an example of this in another companion in Durham, Miriam, about whom I wrote:

> A year ago she had a grown son and daughter; now they are both dead. Her daughter was killed in a car accident in which her son was driving, and six months later her son committed suicide. She is *terribly* sick. She's got such a severe case of diabetes that if she doesn't improve markedly, she may become blind; she has already lost several toes on one foot. In spite of this, she could not stop herself from eating anything and everything containing sugar.
>
> "I was three quarters dead," she told me, "and well on the way to finishing the job off, when suddenly I came out of it—like a parachute opening just when you feel sure you are going to plummet to earth. First of all, I was able to face what I was doing to my husband—the final abandonment of everyone he cared about—but then something even more important happened. I decided that I had to get well in order to find out whether or not I was guilty of the murder of my children. That's how I felt, and I decided that at least there ought to be a *trial*. First I'm going to lick this obesity—and then I'm going to figure out whether or not I have a right to go on living. It all has to *mean something.*"

To go on living after a great crisis often means making dramatic changes in one's life:

I walked home from the Rice House after lunch with a woman who is beautifully slender and about to go home. She had never been heavy until the man she loved was killed in a car accident. She told me: "Ross and I were perfect for each other, but each of us had been married to the wrong person for a long time and there were children to be considered. Just before his death we had decided that we would each have to go through the agony of divorce— there was no other way for us to live. When he died, I knew my marriage could not go on, but I had no one to talk to, no one to lean on. I tried to kill myself—nothing garish like pills or jumping out a window. I gained seventy pounds, got high blood pressure and finally had a mild stroke. When the doctor assured me I would soon succeed in killing myself, that seemed to shock me back to reality. I've been seeing a psychiatrist since I came here, and I think I'm ready to deal with what must be faced. I'm a bright, talented woman and I don't need a man to take care of me. Getting a divorce is for *me*, not in order to marry someone else. I'm scared, but I think I can make it."

If I have learned anything in long years of introspection, it is that life requires a price if we want to be as fully alive as we can be. We need the courage to pursue the truth of our lives and our selves.

However we get there, all problems with obesity have to do with how we feel about ourselves. Feelings of unworthiness, awareness that we are in some way not fulfilling ourselves, can come about in many ways. We assume that everything we experience is related to being *fat* when, in truth, everything we are experiencing is related to being *alive*. This is true for those who have suffered some great shock or loss; getting fat is the symptom through which they are expressing their inner turmoil about the meaning and purpose of their own lives. Before we get thin and stay that way, we have to discover the feelings that interfere with our being most alive. We have a clear choice to make: Do we dare to face our pain, our vulnerability—or do we close ourselves off from what we feel? There was a moment in Durham when it suddenly seemed agonizingly clear to a group of us:

Last night, Margaret, Agnes, Helga and I were sitting in the lobby, talking. Agnes was telling us her feelings about food and hunger; she had been in a concentration camp for two years and emerged, at the end of the war, weighing eighty-two pounds. She is almost bald—she wears a wig all the time—and she lost all her teeth due to malnutrition. The *real* terror of starvation is something most of us know nothing about; Agnes told us how furious she becomes when any of us says, "I'm starving to death."

Billy joined our group, and for the first time, he really opened up and talked about how it feels to weigh over five hundred pounds. We laughed and cried at his description of having to take two first class seats when he flies; about trying to find chairs strong enough to hold him; of the struggle to stand up once he sat down; of the horror and revulsion he felt about himself when he finished a meal of two or three steaks, a loaf of bread, three orders of french fries, and then was still hungry. Helga took his hand and Margaret's eyes filled with tears. I realized what we were doing for each other; here we were—so naked, so vulnerable, opening ourselves to each other, allowing someone else to know about our pain—exploring feelings that we had kept to ourselves because we thought they were too dangerous to face.

Two young men came in the door and walked through the motel lobby to the front desk. They were talking when they came in, but when they noticed all of us sitting together—a group of fat people—they looked shocked and stopped talking. The whole lobby got very quiet. Then, as clear as a bell, we heard one of the young men say, "Hey, what is this? An *animal farm?*"

I felt a sense of outrage. It seemed to me at that terrible moment that it was *us* against *them*, two stupid jerks too insensitive to have any idea about human suffering. I know that this is nonsense; we all experience pain and we all deal with it in whatever way we can—by facing it or denying it or making a joke of it. But I also know that the people who are willing to examine themselves, and who can even allow themselves to be revealed to others, have a very special kind of courage. "Getting in touch with one's feelings" has become such a hackneyed phrase that I hate to use it—and yet that is really what makes life most meaningful. It is what separates the cowards from the courageous, the weak from the strong. It is certainly the key to losing weight permanently.

4

Getting Ready to Lose Weight– By Finding Yourself

The first stage of getting ready to lose weight involves developing a greater understanding of the reasons why we have become fat. But there is more to it than that; readiness also requires the development of new skills in order to continue a process of self-inquiry during and after dieting.

I have found it absolutely crucial to continue trying to keep in touch with my real feelings. What I propose to do in this chapter is to describe the techniques I've developed for this, and to indicate how I continue to use them.

First, it is essential to make up your mind that there is nothing you can find out about yourself, if your allow your feelings to surface, that is bad or dangerous; whatever you discover is merely human—and universal. Like everyone else, you have the potential to be weak and strong, angel and devil, kind and cruel, angry and grateful, selfish and loving, cruel and compassionate.

If you really accept that basic attitude, nothing will frighten you to such a degree that you will have to deny it.

The methods I am going to suggest are these: (1) keep a daily journal; (2) write down all the dreams you can remember and use them for various imaginative exercises; (3) develop your own ways of meditating; (4) use exercises in fantasizing; and (5) write dialogues based on your dreams and writings.

You may be wondering how you can learn to increase your insight if it is something you are not accustomed to doing. It is helpful if one is naturally imaginative and introspective, but I believe that everyone can increase his or her skills at self-examination. Like any other ability, it takes hard work and lots of practice.

I can't teach anyone exactly how to develop powers of introspection, but I can help you learn ways to teach *yourself* to do it. The more you work at it, the easier it will become, and the better you will do it.

Keeping a Journal

The most important first step is to buy a notebook and begin keeping a daily journal in which you write everything that seems important—not so much events, but feelings, or events that bring feelings into play. Do this every day, possibly before going to bed at night. One night it might be two sentences, another night it might be five pages. Write whatever seems natural and comfortable, but the important thing is to keep writing until something surfaces that *feels* important.

It may be helpful if you keep these questions in mind when you start your journal:

1. How do I feel about myself today?
2. How many things did I do that I hated doing—but enjoyed the outcome?

3. Did I comfort myself in any way?
4. Did I punish myself?
5. How did other people treat me today and what did I do, how did I respond? Did they confirm my feelings about myself? Did I let them take advantage of me? Was I more concerned about pleasing others than meeting my own needs? Did their behavior surprise me in any way? Did anyone say anything that sticks in my mind—that seemed to have some special meaning or importance to me?
6. Did I observe anything, did anything happen, did I do anything, that left a deep impression on me?
7. If I were to live this day over, how would I change it, and why?

There is no point in keeping a journal unless it is a genuine conversation with yourself—a confrontation, in which you can learn something about yourself. Let me give an example of two different journal entries about the same event. One might go:

> Vera and I had lunch together at an expensive restaurant. Fortunately, she had invited me! I had chicken Kiev—I just couldn't resist it. I must have gained three pounds. You poke it and rich, creamy butter spurts out. Never had it before, but Vera said it was an experience, and it was.

The other would start out with the above and then go on:

> I wonder why I made the date with Vera when she called. We haven't seen each other in almost a year. I've been dieting well and know it is fatal to go to a gourmet restaurant right now. I don't even like her very much! What made me say yes? She makes me feel dowdy and dumb; she's always dressed perfectly, knows interesting people, etc. This has been the pattern since we were children. She's glamorous, I'm the country mouse; she whistles and I come.
>   Why do I continue to keep up a relationship where I always feel inferior? I think she calls me when she wants

to feel superior and show off. Why do I cooperate? I guess there is still a part of me that agrees with her—that she's done more with her life than I've done with mine. I ate that damned chicken because I was so mad at myself for continuing to allow people to manipulate me, make me feel like a zero person. *I'm not!*

Compulsive eating occurs most frequently when we are feeling depressed—and often when we aren't even conscious of this fact. Depression makes us behave in self-destructive ways because it is almost always associated with feelings of self-hatred.

Usually what happens to me is that first I begin to feel hungry, then I feel restless, then I don't sleep well and begin to feel tired. Being tired makes me twice as hungry. The depression usually leads to feelings of hopelessness and I tend to become extremely lethargic. Now, when this pattern begins, I am alerted to it. After a day or two I start to recognize the signs, and I search for what has initiated the process. In my daily journal, I write down exactly what I am feeling, and describe the events associated with my feelings. I try to become sensitized to everything I do all day, and I record any dreams I have at night. I deliberately tell myself that nothing whatever is to be gained by getting angry at myself; whatever is happening is part of being human and imperfect and vulnerable, and self-condemnation is only going to add to the sense of depression.

We usually get depressed when we are angry at ourselves or at someone else. Depression is more acceptable to us than anger. What I try to do is find out where the anger is coming from. Obviously, it is some kind of anger that I don't want to face—otherwise it wouldn't mask itself as depression. Sometimes I figure out, after a few days of thinking about it, that I'm angry at myself because I am doing things for other people that I don't want to do. For example, it may be that I know my husband is having a hard time with some problem himself, and so I have tried to be especially solicitous and careful in what I do and say. I write about this in my journal and realize that I'm really mad as hell, because waiting on him too much is keeping me from concentrating on my own writing. It is depriving me of attention *I* need. I try to accept my ambivalence; I want to be kind and loving, but since I am human, I become angry instead. I go on behaving responsibly and sensitively because I want to, but the more I let myself experience my anger *on paper* or *in my head*, the less depressed I feel. Here is one example from my journal after I had lost weight:

> All the signs of depression are coming on strong. Hunger, fatigue, not wanting to do anything but stay in bed, and beginning to sneeze a lot as if I'm getting a cold. I am forcing myself to do one thing—and that is to continue to go swimming every day. I know that activity will help me while I figure out what is wrong. I am trying to control what I eat, but if I eat something between meals I try not to scream at myself—I must try to let it go and write down how I am feeling. At the pool today I was watching two young women in their twenties, exercising. Suddenly I felt a wave of great sadness. I wished I had lost the weight when I was young—when my body had greater resilience, and I wouldn't have been left with some sagging, wrinkled flesh. I felt grief-stricken; there was absolutely nothing I could do to change the facts of my life. I hadn't lost the weight until I was fifty-four, and I could not change that. I can never be thin *and young*. After the sadness came terrible anger at myself—*fury* that I didn't have the courage, the character, to do it at twenty or twenty-five. And then I laughed at myself. Here I go again, blaming that poor kid I was. If I could have done it, I would have done it. And I have a few good years left to enjoy it! O.K., I feel sad and I have a right to grieve. I feel angry—and that's all right too: it's only human. I was too frightened, too controlled by neurotic anxiety and self-hatred, to do it when

I was young. Poor me! How sad! But it is a victory *now*—and not to be taken lightly.

I am beginning to feel more energetic. I am not hungry. The depression has passed. I know it will come back, and when it does, I will deal with it again. If I'm lucky, I'll figure it out in a few days. But if it takes me a month or two, I'll still keep working on it.

No matter how well one may succeed in dealing with both the emotional and the physical aspects of overeating, periods of regression are inevitable. These, too, can be dealt with and conquered. That is why learning techniques for self-study and self-understanding are so essential—not only to get to the point of being able to lose weight, but to be ready at all times to deal with new emergencies. Temporary setbacks are part of the process of living and are quite unavoidable; occasional bouts of gluttony and compulsive eating will continue to occur. Unlike the alcoholic, who can give up drinking as a way of dealing with a compulsion (and a physical disability), fat people have no such option; we need food to survive. It is a "habit" we cannot avoid completely. This means that we are in constant contact with food, facing constant temptation, unable to control all aspects of intake at every moment. The slightest use of excess amounts of salt in any food will make me hungry; the smallest increase in carbohydrates will make me crave more sweets; any normal ups and downs in mood can change my choice of what I eat—because eat I must.

Let me describe an experience in a journal entry that helped me to avoid a serious setback in reaction to a recent experience:

I finished the third chapter of this book the day before yesterday, and began looking over my notes for the fourth chapter. I have been living a spartan but satisfying life here alone at the Cape. It is the coldest April any of my neighbors can remember, and this house is like a sieve—not properly insulated at all. At night the wind blows through the bedroom—it sounds like a pack of wolves! But I dress warmly, do some walking—even made arrangements to swim each day at an indoor pool at a nearby motel—and I have been dieting carefully to lose the few pounds I gained last month while traveling.

Yesterday I went to pieces; I began to feel terribly hungry, irritable, restless and uneasy. I had no idea of what was going on. I became terrified that I would go out and eat something I'm not supposed to. I tried taking a walk along the beach, resting, reading. Then I went to the fish store, thinking I might ward off a real regression by buying myself some shrimp or lobster as a gift to myself for working so hard. It didn't work. I finally went out and bought a box of Oreo cookies, and then later I went out and got a meatball hero sandwich. By last night I was frantic; when I went to bed I slept fitfully.

This morning when I'd dragged myself out of bed, I glanced at my dresser. There is a picture of my mother and father taken just a week before my mother died. Both she and my father looked younger and happier than they had for some time; it was my mother's birthday, and she was in a tender, soft mood. The day after the party I left for California and I never saw her alive again. Looking at the picture at six this morning, I suddenly burst into tears, feeling a terrible, piercing sense of loss and loneliness. *I want my mother!* I suddenly realize that I feel terribly guilty about what I have written about my mother, my whole family, in this book. We all loved each other so much— and it seems as if all I have written about is our problems. I have been upset because I'm feeling guilty for seeming to blame so much of my weight problem on my mother and on the *gemütlich*, food-oriented life of my family. The truth is that I loved them all so much and they all loved me so much, and I feel waves of psychological hunger to go back to childhood—to bring them all back to life, to relive it all. There it is again: guilt and ambivalence, it gets me every time. Today—nothing but fruit juices!

Writing something down and then reading it makes it seem more benign—no matter how intense the original feelings may have been. We give up hope if we think that an eating binge can't be stopped. Writing about it helps to slow it down. After forty-eight hours of panic, I was steady again. All was *not* lost. I could now go back to work and dieting. I could live with my mixed feelings; I knew they were normal and that I could accept the pain of being human. For the moment, I was back on an even keel. There is a sense of relief and release, a catharsis, in writing and then reading what one has written.

Keeping a journal is simply a way of having a discussion with oneself. Here are some further examples that I think indicate the process that takes place:

I feel lousy. I think I have the flu. I'm hungry all the time, in spite of feeling sick. Some sort of primitive feeling seems close to the surface: *What is it?* I know it has to do with the fact that I've lost weight. Getting thin and getting sick. Ah, I think I've got it: deep inside me is a voice saying, "If you don't eat, you'll get sick." The childhood equation. God, it's so strong. But I must tell myself it is *irrational.*

Yesterday I went crazy—the first really compulsive eating of all kinds of junk since I came home from Durham. Couldn't stop myself. The old pattern returned in full force, and I couldn't figure out what was happening to me. I realize this morning that I've been pushing myself much too hard— trying to get a children's book finished, having constant company, trying to meet everyone's needs but my own. The reason I was able to break the pattern in Durham was that nobody could get at me; I was doing only what I wanted to do, with no demands from anyone. It is a thousand times harder at home. Under the pressure of "real life," it is so easy to retreat into old, familiar patterns of handling fatigue, frustration, anger. Food is still a way in which I avoid facing those kinds of feelings. The only difference is that now I am more sensitized to it, and I do something about it more quickly. I stayed in bed most of today, just resting and reading. Screw the rest of the world! I don't have to be Mother Earth—people will just have to get off my back and leave me alone. I didn't clean the house, I let all the "shoulds" go—even getting exercise. I knew I had to let go completely, crawl into a cocoon and shut the world out.

I didn't know I was going to do it, but I seem to have put myself back on rice and fruit. The impulse toward health is stronger now than the impulse toward self-destruction. Maybe all one can do is shift the balance. Nobody ever overcame self-destructive feelings altogether; you just shift the balance on the side of life!

Keeping a journal in which you get in touch with your feelings is a way of becoming your own most important friend.

Recording Your Dreams

One important use for your journal is to record all the dreams you can remember. Talk to yourself about them on paper. It is likely that if you don't ordinarily remember your dreams, it may take some days or weeks of recording your thoughts before you can begin to recall enough details. Keep a pad and pencil next to your bed and try to write your dreams down the minute you wake up; otherwise you are likely to forget them. But don't get angry at yourself if at first you can't remember. This means you are not ready, and getting angry at yourself is precisely the wrong reaction. Getting in touch with one's feelings is possible only in an atmosphere of love, self-acceptance and patience.

Understanding one's dreams is a skill that improves with practice, and you can develop this ability as you go along. There are as many ways to interpret dreams as there are schools of psychotherapy, but what I discovered over the years was that even though individual therapists might have different approaches, each came to the same general conclusions as to the basic feelings and themes reflected in my dreams. Each of us develops a special style and a unique language. When I dream of being in a basement or downstairs, it usually means I'm dealing with deeply buried, unconscious material. Dreaming about the brownstone house in which I lived as a young child means I'm involved in very early childhood experiences. Dreaming of water or travel or a bridge means that I am coming to a new place in my development—traveling into new territory. When I dream about various rooms in a house, the rooms usually represent different parts of myself. Dreaming about Nazi storm troopers means that I am dreaming about how much I hate myself, what an evil person I think I am. You will find that slowly but surely, themes tend to repeat themselves and become familiar.

The work of dreams goes on even when we can't remember them; then they sometimes help us to solve problems at an unconscious level. The importance of remembering dreams and trying to understand what they mean to us is that they can help us grow and change. And besides, it's so interesting. Dreams help us to discover how adorable we really are! Our minds are so much more creative, funny, sweet, charming than we give them credit for being!

Here are some clues to help you to begin to understand your dreams:

1. Some dreams are wish fulfillments—the hungry man dreaming of food, the repressed lady who dreams of a man hiding under her bed!
2. Dreams are ways of expressing feelings you might not dare to express in your conscious life. If you tend to be placid, easygoing, good-natured, and your dreams are full of bloodthirsty violence, there is a split between two normal parts of yourself that need reconnecting, now that you are an adult

and know that there is no such thing as being all good or all bad. We are all a mixture of both and that is not dangerous because we can control our *behavior;* it is not necessary or even healthy to repress and control all our *thoughts.* It works the other way too. People who drive themselves to the point of total psychic exhaustion may have calm, quiet, bucolic dreams.

3. All the characters in any dream relate to parts of yourself in addition to possibly representing other people. After all, it's your dream, and the people are your invention. For example, you might dream about your father in a situation where he is making you very angry because he is being aggressive and punitive. Possibly this really was a quality of your father (or in your feelings about him), but it could also reflect the fact that you feel you have some of that same quality in yourself and you don't like it.

4. Dreams can be used as springboards to exploration of an experience. If there are two characters in the dream, you could continue the drama after awakening by writing a dialogue between them, to see where they take you. Or you might write the continuation of the dream as an ongoing story. You could choose one person in your dream and construct a conversation between the two of you. Or take a character in a dream who seems vague, mysterious, confusing, and sit down and write his or her case history.

5. Very often, when we are dreaming about a very deep and primitive part of ourselves, we tend to be the opposite sex. One theory about this occurrence is that each of us has within us some of the characteristics of the other sex—both physically and psychologically—and the unconscious sees this as a shadow side of ourselves.

The thing to remember about understanding your dreams is that there are no right or wrong answers. It's your dream and you can do whatever you want with it. It is true that a skilled therapist might help you to see things you otherwise might miss, but the important thing is not the dream itself but the process through which you are trying to gain access to more and more parts of yourself. The dream is just a tool—a point of departure. It's the process of exploration that is important—thinking, feeling, contemplating. Using the dream as the basis of a daydream, for example, is simply a technique for discovering more about yourself. We tend to be too lugubrious about dreams—to take them too seriously. Don't be intimidated.

Dreams are another form of a conversation with oneself. They need demystification. Be *playful* with your dreams. There is no reason to be afraid of doing this, because if you are not ready to figure something out, you just won't be able to do it.

Here are some examples of the ways in which I have used my dreams for greater self-understanding:

1. Dealing with Fears

I dream I am in a big house, where there are lots of people, lots of activity. At first I don't want to get involved with cooking—I want to get dressed up and go to parties. I begin to think it is Christmas time and that my mother died several years ago. But then I have the feeling this will be the first Christmas without my father too, and I feel very sad and upset—and then I get involved with the cooking. Now it is a brownstone house—very busy, very pressured. I am getting tense and tired, but then realize that both my parents are sitting on the couch, looking very happy and smiling at me. They are alive and well, after all.

My interpretation of the dream is that when I want to forget about eating and food and change my priorities, I lose my parents—my childhood, really. When I return to a preoccupation with food, I recapture my parents and my childhood. That

brownstone house of my grandparents, where food and cooking
and eating were the focus around which we all lived, was a
place of safety and security and love. I'm afraid if I give up
that pattern, I have to lose the people and the memories. *I don't!*
That's just my irrational unconscious acting up again.

2. *Dealing with Anger*

I dream that I am in a large hotel ballroom, with space
for three thousand people, but I am there all alone and
every table is loaded with food. I finish all the food at one
table and go on to the next. Realize in the dream that if I
keep on doing this I will become monstrously fat—worse
than ever before—but I can't stop myself.

Wake up in a cold sweat—terrified. As I lie in bed trying
to think, introspect, about what is going on right now, it
occurs to me that maybe I'm mad at myself because of that
damned speech I promised to give. I have avoided my professional role so carefully since coming to Durham—this is
my time for *me*—and yet I let myself get talked into doing
it. I think I'm angry at that part of me that still gives in,
that doesn't protect me from this invasion by the "real
world" when I'm not ready yet. The anger against myself
is what makes me want myself fat again, the terrible punishment. I have to be a watchdog—ever alert for the things I
do that I don't want to do that make me angry at myself.

3. *Dealing with Anxieties about Dieting*

I dream that an old friend (younger, very slim, an artist)
is in church with her son. She's very busy serving food
and doesn't notice me at all. Someone hands me a letter,
which says, "It's wonderful to hear you now weigh 250
pounds." I am horrified—terrified. My God, did I get fatter

instead of thinner? I feel a sense of relief when I realize I don't know the person who sent the letter.

It seems to me that the dream is telling me that my unconscious mind is just as preoccupied with my dieting as I know I am consciously. There is the preoccupation with food, the anxiety, the ambivalence about losing weight. The letter was expressing my anxiety about whether or not I am going to succeed. The person the letter came from was really myself, but it was too painful to know I could be so mixed up and so I changed it to a stranger.

4. The Dream As a Warning

I dream that it is snowy, miserable weather. I am having a great deal of trouble maneuvering from place to place. I seem to have moved and nothing is where it is supposed to be. The refrigerator is in a deep hole and I can only open the door partway. I think my boots are in there but I can't get at them and am becoming frantic. Wendy and Nancy (both beautiful and glamorous) and I are supposed to be going to the opera. The two of them are dressed in original, flamboyant, gorgeous dresses. I am stuck with all this disorder and confusion, which seems at the moment to center around my problems with the refrigerator. I feel terribly angry, frustrated and hopeless.

This dream occurred during Christmas week. When I woke up, my first thought was: This is my first *thin* Christmas! I have been getting up at 5:30 A.M. every day to work on this book; Larry is out of town at a three-week seminar. I told everyone to leave me alone to work—no parties, no fun. Larry and I had agreed we would both work hard during the holiday season because we are going to take a vacation in February, but I feel bitchy and I've been eating too much.

The dream begins to help me see what is happening. In the dream everything is disorganized, and unpleasant—except that in the background are those two beautiful, glamorous women all dressed up and ready to go out. I am trying to get to the refrigerator, which is full of all kinds of things in total disorder—which is unlike me! I wrote in my journal:

> I am really very upset—even angry—that my first "thin Christmas" is being spent in this isolation chamber. The book is the refrigerator, all confused, all about food. Nowhere to go, no one to get dressed up for. This has been entirely my own choice—but if I want to have ambivalent feelings about it, why shouldn't I?
>
> I went to bed last night exhausted and depressed because I just could not imagine how all my disorganized notes could ever turn into a book. I'll have to just sit here, and try to figure it out. *But I'm really mad!* I want to get dressed up in my new clothes and go out, looking very glamorous! If I don't want to start eating too much, I'd better call a friend and get some theater or opera tickets, and not work quite so hard.

5. Using a Dream for a Dialogue with Oneself

Last night I dreamed I was decorating a new house. I woke up feeling wonderful. It was a happy, satisfying dream and I knew at once the house was myself. I decided that this might be a good time, while I'm feeling good, to write a dialogue between my selves, looking back at how I felt about coming to Durham.

EDA 1: They will laugh at me.

EDA 2: You are a grown woman, nobody laughs at you anymore. That was when you were a little girl.

EDA 1: I'm too ashamed. I'm shy.

EDA 2: No, you are full of the *memory* of feeling that way.

Actually, you are quite poised and self-assured. People respect and like you.

EDA 1: I won't have the strength of character.

EDA 2: We will have to wait and see about that.

The dream seems to suggest I'm making it!

6. The Dream as the Beginning of a Story

Another useful "game" is to take a character that may appear and reappear in your dreams but somehow always remains vague and mysterious, and write a description of him or her. Often in my dreams there is a young boy, somewhere between seven and fourteen years old. He seems to sort of flit by or be in the background. I never could "catch" him, so I wrote the following description:

THE BOY

He is tall and skinny and very active physically—he's always moving. Wears torn dungarees and a T-shirt and old, torn sneakers. He moves with the gracefulness of a leopard. Lives at the sea, spends much time around docks and boats and looking at sea gulls and talking to fishermen. Sort of half boy, half girl, young adolescent in general—but very wise. Likes bicycling, swimming, walking, but even though he likes to be moving, he can be very steady and slow and quiet some of the time. Quiet inner rhythm about him.

A very "inside" person. Shy, doesn't care to talk much, likes to observe others. Is going to be a writer. A deep, quiet passion for it. Doesn't need other people very much, lives inside himself a great deal of the time. But can be loving and warm to a few people. Feels no sense of rush about anything, just takes the moment and doesn't plan ahead. Has no great need or desire to go anywhere or accomplish anything. Loves flowers and gardening. Hardly ever eats at all, can forget all about it for days at a time. But when he does eat he enjoys it—briefly but well.

Once I had got this down on paper, it was completely transparent: *I* want to be like that boy—I already am, in part, for I dreamed him. In my dreams he is a kind of background music to remind me how differently I actually live—often doing severe damage to this necessary inner self. It has been helpful to think about this boy—to know he is there.

7. *Having Fun with Dreams*

I dream that Larry is very upset because of electrical overloading in the apartment. He says we ought to be causing short circuits all the time—he doesn't understand why this isn't happening.

As I woke up, it occurred to me that working on this book is a heavy emotional load because I have been trying to deal with the past and the present simultaneously—and I'm afraid I'll blow a fuse!

8. *The Dream As Enrichment—a Path for Growing*

I dream I am in a rambling, big, attractive summer home—like a small English estate or a French chateau. I realize there are many more rooms than I have ever been aware of, many as yet unexplored. I open a door, go up some steps, feel very excited to discover all kinds of new treasures I never knew were there. Then I come back to a central area and discover a gorgeous bed of flowers, wild, sensual, some tropical—I'd never imagined there was such a place. Larry tells me he ordered the flowers to be put there and the workmen are just finishing the garden. I am very surprised.

There are lots of merry children in the garden. The whole scene is relaxed, casual, happy. The next morning a friend arrives with some new clothes for me to try on. The blouses I choose are so elegant! Can that really be *me?*

Later, as I thought about the dream, I realized there are wonderful unexplored areas of living and feeling—unexplored territories in my own head (the house). I realized that Larry and I are both changing and that this is nothing to fear, nothing to feel guilty about. This time my unconscious was willing to take a chance on it all working out all right!

Using your dreams in all these ways can help you to realize more of your potential in all aspects of your life—but only if you do it without any sense of pressure. Under these circumstances dreams can be a means of enriching your life experience, adding a new dimension to the ways in which you explore yourself and your environment.

Learning to Meditate

Something that has made a great difference to me in recent years—and added immeasurably to my ability to deal with my feelings—has been learning to meditate. Meditation had become a great interest of my husband's, and at first I joined some of his training seminars just to find out what it was he was teaching. I stayed to discover that meditation is an exceedingly helpful way to get in touch with one's feelings. He happens to have written a dandy book on the subject,* and since I am not an expert, I am not going to discuss it in any detail—except to say that if *I* could learn to meditate, anyone can! It came as a great shock to discover that if I really worked at it, I could indeed achieve short periods in which I did absolutely nothing but the one thing I'd set myself to do—meditate. Our minds tend to be wildly undisciplined, and if you lead as active and hectic a life as I usually do, the ability to call a halt and take time alone can enable you to heal your mental fractures as you focus your thoughts on what you feel is really important. I highly

* Lawrence LeShan, *How to Meditate* (Boston: Little, Brown, 1974; Bantam ed., 1975).

recommend training courses in meditation, with the warning that if such programs cost a great deal of money, if they have a Madison Avenue slickness in packaging and promotion, and if they promise all sorts of wonders—run, do not walk, to the nearest exit.

Learning to meditate is *not* the same as free associating. It is a very tough mental discipline, but one that is "natural" for human beings. Its naturalness can be seen in two ways: first, a good session of work at it makes you feel "put together" and whole; and second, it has been invented and reinvented over and over again in the history of the human race. Every period of history and every society we know about has found some special exercises or rituals to help people go into a meditative or prayerful state of mind. The best books and courses on meditation are those in which the authors have sifted through the thousands of meditational exercises now available and chosen the ones that seem most understandable and relevant in our culture.

There is great value to one's entire mental and physical well-being in learning to be still and totally focused, even if you can do it for only a few seconds at a time. That simple accomplishment is remarkable enough; all the gobbledegook about mysterious and mystical rewards (such as being able to levitate) are just sensationalism and advertising techniques. The true practitioners who spend their lives trying to achieve the perfect state make far fewer claims than do many entrepreneurs now offering all kinds of "mind trips." I have found meditation a way in which to experience an inner peace and tranquillity, a way of becoming less fragmented. There is no question that such feelings can be very helpful during the stressful periods of getting ready to diet, dieting, and adjusting to being thinner.

Exercise Your Fantasies

There are some excellent books that offer exercises to aid you in making up your own fantasies. One that I have found especially helpful is *Mind Games* by Jean Houston (Dell). There are also a number of workshops now being offered that are designed to help you learn how to study yourself through your own fantasies. But be careful not to choose the ones that are strictly commercial enterprises.

Let me try to give you some idea of how this fantasizing process can work. You can make up all kinds of situations on your own, and the more unique and individual they are, the more useful they will be. Here are some examples:

1. Once every six months or so, I ask myself what I would do if I had only six more months to live. If I determine that I would want to change my life in any major way, then I am living someone else's life, not my own. The question helps to remind me of what my real priorities are and where I may have been losing my way.

2. A similar question is: "If this were my birthday and I was *really* my own best friend, what would I give myself?" People have reported to me that they are sometimes quite astounded by their spontaneous responses—ranging from a course in ceramics to a trip around the world or a day at the beach or a pet kitten. When you analyze the qualities in the gift you first thought of, you will know something more about your needs.

3. Sit down in a comfortable chair and imagine that there is a giant movie screen in front of you and you can make up the movie of the rest of your life—or some part of it, maybe the next year or two. What images come to mind? What can you learn about your innermost wishes and needs? For a while the "screen" may remain blank, but if you can relax and be patient, without forcing anything, you will probably soon begin to "see" things that may be more important to you than you ever knew before.

4. Make up the beginning of a story that leads to travel. One could be: "I see this strange old castle and I go inside and

see a winding staircase. I walk down and find myself at a
small underground lake. There is a rowboat tied to the wall.
I get in and row away. . . ." Or: "I'm on the edge of a forest.
The trees are dense and it is all strange and unfamiliar, but
I decide to explore the woods. I think it may get dark before
I can find my way out, but I make up my mind I will sleep
in the woods if necessary. . . ." Or: "I meet a group of children playing and begin to talk to them. They are all different
ages, but they seem to be related to one another. They ask
me to take them on a trip and I decide we will go. . . ."

All I am doing, really, is setting up situations in which you
are required to make decisions about what you are going to
do with your life. When you first try these exercises they may
seem like a waste of time—child's play. The truth is that child's
play is just about the most important thing any child ever does;
it is the way he discovers himself. In a sense, I am inviting
you to go back to a time in your life when your imagination
helped you to discover your needs and feelings.

The first few times you make up these fantasies or write them
down as stories, they may seem dull and repetitious—even silly
and embarrassing—but remember that you are not showing
them to anyone else, and after a while you will be amazed to
discover how certain themes seem to be repeated over and over
again. Let me give some personal examples:

> I get to the bottom of the steps but I have a terrible time
> trying to untie the rowboat. Someone has left it with a
> complicated and difficult knot. At first I feel hopeless—I
> will never get the boat loose—but I rest awhile and then
> try again. Finally I get it loose but I am too worn out,
> too tired to row, so I just let the boat float along on its
> own. I come to a kind of marshland where all the colors
> are pastel—pinks, yellows, very light greens, blues, very
> quiet and peaceful. There are a few very large birds, like

herons and sea gulls, but they don't make a sound and they fly in slow motion. The place makes me so sleepy that I am afraid I will stop breathing. I force myself to start rowing. My heart beats wildly and I get all out of breath. I want to stay there, but I'm afraid that if I let myself go, I'll never get back.

If I got lost in the woods, I would become very drowsy and fall asleep—which could be very dangerous since there probably are wild animals lurking there to kill me. But I have no choice; the woods are so peaceful and quiet I just cannot keep walking. Maybe I could climb a tree and find a safe branch where I could curl up and sleep. In the morning I will find a family of pandas, all looking at me in a very friendly and loving way. I could stay with them.

On the movie screen all I can seem to see is chaos—subways rushing and screeching, taxis honking, planes taking off, blasting their pollution right off the screen and at me. No matter how I try, I can't change the image. When there begins to be rock music, I cover my ears and feel very depressed.

These fantasies occurred several years ago. I had returned home after an exhausting publicity tour for one of my books that had been overscheduled in every city. Every fantasy centered around my need to let go, become dependent and rest—but each time there was some anxiety about doing this. My thoughts were a reminder that I simply *had* to take time to rest. Even more than providing insight, the fantasies were comforting and pleasurable; in themselves, they were giving me some of the relaxation I needed.

Having Dialogues with Yourself

Making up conversations between yourself and dream characters or real people who seem to have a great influence on your feelings

is another technique to broaden and deepen your self-explorations. It can be fun—as well as revealing. For example, many
years ago I dreamed about Pearl Bailey three times in one week
and could not figure out why—until I made up the following
dialogue:

EDA: Pearl, why do I keep dreaming about you?

PEARL: Honey, if *you* don't know, how am I supposed to
figure it out?

EDA: I've been trying to. I seem to remember that you had
a bad heart attack, that you lost a lot of weight, and that
you looked wonderful the next time I saw you on TV.
How can you go on working so hard after a heart attack?
Where do you get so much energy?

PEARL: Honey, I'm just *doing my thing*. How can a person
get sick or tired if every day they are doing what makes
them happy?

EDA: Didn't you feel funny when you lost all that weight?
I mean, weren't you afraid that when you got thin you'd
be somebody else?

PEARL: Listen—I was so sick and so scared, and if you know
you're gonna die you just don't worry about such things.
I felt marvelous when I got skinny.

EDA: What is the matter with me? Why can't I stick to a
diet? I get so hungry and then I stuff myself. I can't stop
and I don't understand it.

PEARL: Well, I suppose it's harder to go through it unless
you have to, like I did. Dieting is no damn fun. I *love*
food. Now I'm just too busy to want to eat.

EDA: I wonder if it would help me diet if I had your feeling
that I was really "doing my thing"? I almost never feel
that way. Last summer, writing the children's book, I
felt really good; also making that TV series—but now,
almost never. Lately I've been running around giving
speeches—and getting fatter. I feel miserable.

PEARL: Honey, I can *see* you are in *trouble!*

EDA: I wish you could tell me what to do. If you can't, why do I keep dreaming you?

PEARL: Maybe you dream me to remind you what life could be like if you just got down to business and got it over with.

EDA: I keep feeling I mustn't do it.

PEARL: Why, for heaven's sake?

EDA: I just don't know. I get very frightened that something awful will happen to me. I *know* it's crazy.

PEARL: What you got to feel so guilty about, that you can't let yourself be happy and pretty?

EDA: I don't know, I don't know!

PEARL: You got some kind of hangup that you just got to look fat? Or you just got to hide that you got as much energy as me?

EDA: I'm all mixed up.

PEARL: Well, honey, you dreamed me, so I must be part of you—and you *know* you like me!

EDA: Yes, I do! I love watching you. You seem so at home in the world, so full of love, so happy to be doing what you do. I'd like to be like you—

PEARL: Then what's stopping you?

EDA: Because you are being your *real self*—and somehow I feel that's dangerous and bad.

PEARL: You look like a pretty old girl to me! Almost fifty years old! When you gonna start deciding what you want to do with your life, for heaven's sake?

EDA: We're getting nowhere. I still don't know why I can't diet, or why I dream about you, and why I can't write anymore.

PEARL: You certainly don't sound happy about your work. That's bad, real bad.

EDA: I don't want to write books that lecture *at* people anymore. I want to write my innermost feelings—maybe even try fiction. I'm sick and tired of being an "expert"—

PEARL: Honey, I think maybe you hit it! You want to express

yourself, just for your own pleasure, not to teach other
people. Maybe—

EDA: But a good novelist teaches other people a lot.

PEARL: But that ain't what he sets out to do. He just has
to write what's in his heart, no matter what. When you
write, you *know* you are trying to give lessons, and that
doesn't please you *at all*.

EDA: Lecturing people on how to live instead of just living.

PEARL: Honey, that's what it's *all* about!

This dialogue lets me quickly verbalize the two parts of myself—the part that feels caught in a web of doing what is expected
of me (and what I expect of myself) and the other part, trying
to get free of the "shoulds." I see that the earthy, humorous
part is the self that I need to get better acquainted with. Now
it is someone I have no contact with, a famous star, whom I've
never met; the dialogue makes me want to meet that person
inside me. Since I wrote that dialogue, slowly but surely my
books have become less didactic, more personal.

Sometimes we dream of a character we just cannot stand, a
person we loathe with a passion. I assume, when this happens
to me, that it is a part of myself that I don't want to have anything
to do with—and therefore one that's important to confront.

In one such dream of mine, her name is Muriel and she is
horrible! I hate and fear her. She embodies all the things I dislike
most: she's puritanical, authoritarian, rigid. Most of all, she
makes me hate myself—she makes me depressed and hungry,
fills me with self-loathing. I feel as if Muriel's whole purpose
in "life" is to make me feel old and fat and ugly. It would be
impossible to have any direct relationship with her. Florence
(my therapist) wants me to have a dialogue with her. I hate
the idea, but I'll try.

The following is just a sample from a much longer dialogue:

E. I really don't want to stop eating to write this stupid
thing. I just want to sink into an abyss of self-pity and

misery. I have no desire to talk to you at all.

M. That's fine with me; just the way I like things.

E. Why are you so evil?

M. I am whatever you let me be.

E. I am absolutely miserable.

M. What makes you think that I'm not?

E. Could you at least try to tell me why you are unhappy too?

M. Because you have assigned me a completely impossible role. One-dimensional, inhuman, all bad. Because you are so frightened of your real feelings that you have made me into the most terrible policeman. You have made me into a snarling watchdog that must be on guard every second of the day and night. Why aren't you willing to accept Florence's offer to mediate between us? I was really hoping you'd bring her into this conversation.

E. All right. Talk to Florence.

F. Muriel, I'd like to intervene. I know you have been suffering, but I find it very hard to help Eda to see that.

M. For a moment there in your office today, I thought you had helped to break through when she said I was a child.

E. Yes, I feel that maybe Muriel is something I created when I was a little girl, and that there is something sad about the burdens I gave her.

F. Oh, Eda, don't stop there. *What* burdens did you give her? Why *did* you create her?

E. Because I was so bad, because I just couldn't be good, because I was so damned scared—

F. What were you scared of?

E. The things I would do.

F. *What?*

E. I hardly know. The Nazi in me, the whore, the murderer, the liar, the thief.

F. Eda, right now you can tell *me* what you want to say to Muriel—what you have wanted to say to her for many, many years.

E. Muriel, I'm not bad. I want to be free, and alive. I want to feel things, to experience my life fully—and I'm not bad. You don't have to watch me so much any more.

M. Florence, she still doesn't understand, does she? Eda, I can't stop watching over you until you let us *both* live a little. You are part of me, I am part of you.

E. You mean that I've got to homogenize myself?

F. Something like that.

E. One must carry one's freight of childhood, mustn't one? There is no alternative. I cannot kick out either side, any piece of it—I have to learn to tolerate the complexity of me.

M. That's called integration, you idiot.

E. We are so torn and weary and afraid and unalive, the way we are—I can't bear it anymore.

M. Neither can I. Take pity on me, Eda, please. I am suffering too.

E. I'm trying. The bad girl won't leave.

F. Don't try to make her leave—

M. We could take care of her together.

E. That's *it!* That's *it!* We are her *parents*—together! We have to learn to let her breathe.

M. Yes! Yes! That's all I ever really wanted. To be a parent, and to help you do the best you could. I don't want to be a torturer.

E. I am a good girl and a bad girl; I'm everything. I have to live with the danger, don't I?

F. I think you're getting there.

This dialogue was greatly enhanced when I was able to comfort myself by bringing my therapist into the game. What I was struggling about was a universal human problem. When we are young and we do something naughty, someone usually says, "Now, *that* wasn't the *good* little Janey that did that—there must be a *bad* little Janey somewhere around." Wanting to please the people we love and who love us, we unconsciously split ourselves in two. We create a policeman to guard over our impulses, our creativity, our vitality—because those are qualities that can get you into trouble, make grownups angry. As adults, we need to face the fact that those are also the best parts of ourselves and that we have the maturity to control our behavior and make choices. The "bad child" and the "good child" need to be reintegrated if we are to become whole.

Getting Help

If you find that trying the various exercises I've described above simply leads to greater confusion and anxiety, then it seems to me your only alternative is to seek guidance and counseling of some kind. Sometimes the fears—the psychic damage—have been so crippling that one cannot explore oneself without the aid and comfort of someone who understands the process and can help one feel safe enough to face the necessary exploration that can lead to change and growth. I hope that if after reading this book you feel you need further help, you will have the courage to seek other resources.*

If you are choosing a therapist, it is extremely important to do it carefully, for unless the therapist represents a point of view and an approach that suit your special needs and your own sense of values, therapy is not likely to be of any help to you.

A friend of mine, after beginning to work with a particular psychiatrist, called me, and in a breathless and hopeful tone of voice said, "He isn't trying to *change* me—he just wants to help me to be *myself!*" If I had to pick one useful criterion for choosing a therapist, that would be it—someone who can help you search for your own unique strengths.

* I've written on this subject in my book *The Wonderful Crisis of Middle Age*, (New York: David McKay, 1973; Warner paperback, 1974), Chapter 7, "The Heavy Burden of Our Masks"; and "Therapy: Can it Help?" *Woman's Day Magazine*, March 1978.

Therapy, at its best, is a technique for exploring "internal roots." It is a method for searching for the child you once were, and for setting some things straight. It ought to represent a time and a place where you feel safe to explore old and new feelings. A good therapist is a companion on a journey.

Here are some fundamental questions for you to ask when you're searching for the right kind of help. First of all, has this person done his homework? Has he studied all the various schools of psychotherapy and does he now bring special creativity to this background knowledge? Is he a flexible person, able to admit uncertainty and mistakes? Does this person have a philosophy of life that is similar to your own? Do you feel an immediate rapport? Is it easy to begin to say what you feel, knowing that he will be totally honest in his reactions? Does the therapist seem to care genuinely about you, as a person? Is as much attention given to your strengths and possibilities as to the ways in which you may have lost your way? And most important of all, is this someone you can like so much that you might very well have chosen him for a friend?

It has been my experience that the particular professional title is less significant than the individual. There are wonderful psychiatrists, psychologists, social workers and family counselors—and there are awful ones. No profession is immune from the wide range of talent and integrity one sees among people in general. It is important to trust your own judgment, and to keep on looking until you feel you have found someone you can work with.

Each of us has his own special ways of learning and growing. Some of us do our best introspection in a one-to-one relationship; others may find a group experience exciting and enlightening. Some people just need a kind of "booster shot"—a few sessions of counseling—while others may feel they want to take the time and make the effort to do some long-term explorations. There are types of therapy to suit all such needs, and a first step in considering the possibility of therapy is to find out about the various resources in your community.

Psychotherapy can be expensive—but here again, there are alternatives. Many therapists have a sliding scale of fees, and this will certainly be true of social agencies; often medical insurance coverage includes psychotherapy. Finances are most assuredly a factor to be considered, but this should never be the deciding factor in choosing a therapist. A less expensive therapist whom you don't really like compared with an expensive one whom you are crazy about should involve no conflict at all. There are always ways to pay the cost of therapy over a long period of time, or to borrow money, if necessary. Therapy is too important a process for you to look for bargains.

Trusting one's instincts is a valid approach in choosing a therapist, for you will be dealing with feelings all through the process—and that's a good way to begin. If you make a mistake in judgment, you can try someone else. It's a painful and often difficult process, but one well worth pursuing.

One word of caution: Run, do not walk, to the nearest exit if any therapist assures you he or she has all the answers and can easily or quickly solve all your problems. *Life* is full of problems and always will be. Therapy can only help you meet those problems more effectively.

During my adolescence, a factor that surely did not help me deal with the problem of obesity was the fact that our family doctor was (in addition to really caring deeply about me) a highly neurotic man, driven by his own inner demons. Every visit to his office included The Lecture: I would ruin my whole life if I did not diet. If I didn't solve this problem I would be subject to terrible diseases. Didn't I want to be attractive? I could be a very pretty girl if only . . . Every year it would get harder and harder to lose weight; he knew I was cheating—if I dieted as he instructed me to, there would be no problem.

I was sure that he wanted the best for me and that I was some kind of monster because I could not measure up to his expectations. However, I also recall his affection, his genuine concern when I was seriously ill. He used to write me letters to cheer me up when I was sick, or away at camp, and every letter ended with, "May your shadow grow less." It was a joke between us—that if I got thinner, I'd have a smaller shadow.

Many years later, influenced by the theories of Carl Jung, I came to have a special understanding of "my shadow." It was the part of myself that was unconscious; the part I had not been able to accept, the source of my creativity and drive, but buried too long in fear—hidden as something "bad."

The doctor could not have imagined that the way I would cause my shadow to grow less would be not only by getting thinner, but also by learning to accept my shadow, enjoy it, use it. I am no longer threatened by my shadow, do not see it as some terrible enemy to be kept at bay at all costs. My shadow and I have become one.

May *your* shadow grow less ominous to you as you, too, begin the long, hard road to getting in touch with the side of yourself that you have not yet acknowledged, but which will present itself to you as you start talking to yourself. There is nothing to fear from one's shadow; it is a source of splendid human qualities.

5

Choosing
a Diet
Is Like Getting
Married

The choice of a specific diet is of infinite importance. As in choosing a spouse, it ought to be for better, for worse, in sickness and in health—and to some degree at least, it will probably be part of your life forever.

Getting ready to make this choice is a gradual process. You will *not* wake up one morning and discover you are ready to diet, that you have straightened yourself out, are now neurosis-free and know exactly what you want to do. What will happen is that over a period of time in the course of your self-explorations you will begin to sense that you no longer really need to be fat.

I believe that *any* diet will work if you are ready and if it happens to suit you as an individual. The best and most sensible way to diet is to go to your family doctor, get a nice, well-balanced 600- or 800-calorie-a-day diet, and stay on it with religious fervor until you are the right weight. That's a terrific idea for someone who needs to lose five or ten pounds. For those of us who have to lose any amount above, say, twenty pounds, the likelihood of our staying on that kind of diet is very slim (!) indeed. We feel so overwhelmed by the long process involved that we are discouraged before we begin. This is, of course, the source of the fascination with quick fad diets. As a matter of fact, if you are really obese and have developed serious diseases in conjunction with the overweight, many doctors will agree that the 600- to 800-calorie diet is too slow a process.

All kinds of seemingly crazy diets become faddish, and apparently the human body can stand almost any diet for a while; but there can be very serious aftereffects if such a diet is continued over a long period of time. There are people who have eaten chicken legs and vitamins for a month; there are people who have lived on coffee and fruit juice even longer—and they seem to be able to recover their health and be well nourished afterward. However, nobody can or should try to stay on a fad diet indefinitely. *I am in no position ethically or medically to offer any suggestions about the type of diet you ought to go on.* It may take you months or even years to hit on the diet that is right for you, and you will just have to keep experimenting until you know you have found it. I *can* tell you what happened to me—not to endorse the specific program that worked for me, but to show you the sort of process you will more than likely have to go through. Do not for one moment assume that my solution is your solution. *It must be your own.* Each of us has her own unique biology, her physiological reactions to certain foods, and because so little is yet known about this, one has no choice but to trust one's own instincts.

What happens to most of us is that we try *everything.* Each diet works for a short period of time, then fails, and we blame ourselves. We tell ourselves that if we were mature, self-controlled people, the diet would work. I have come to the conclusion that this is nonsense. When I found the right diet for me—the one that had every characteristic I needed—I lost weight very quickly. Even though I was psychologically ready for some time before that, I had not been able to lose weight quickly enough to feel encouraged on other diets. To find the diet that's right for you, it's important to find: (1) the right medical personnel; (2) the right group to diet with (such as Weight Watchers or Overeaters Anonymous), unless you decide you are the kind of person who prefers to do it privately; (3) the right environment in which to diet; and (4) the diet that *feels right*. This last point is important: Does your body feel as if what you are doing is what you have been waiting for all your life? As you become sensitized and more in tune with your emotions, you will become more aware of the nuances of your physical well-being as well.

Does the diet make you feel good? Do you lose quickly enough to make you want to stick with it? This is important not only during the period of dieting; the right diet is one that you will be able to live with, to a lesser degree, for the rest of your life.

Don't be impatient if it takes a long time to find the diet that is perfect for you. It may require a great deal of experimentation. As soon as you go off a diet, don't berate yourself for being a rotten person; assume that the diet just wasn't built to suit your unique and special needs.

Choosing a Doctor and a Program

Among the fifteen to twenty of those from whom I sought help, I cannot recall a single doctor who did not make me feel guilty when I failed. To some degree, I think this attitude also exists in the various group programs. If it isn't overt, it is at least present as a subtle and unconscious demand. After all, our failure is seen as an attack on the doctor or the group; this seems to be a given that we simply have to put up with—and ignore.

The program that finally worked for me was run by a man with a religious fervor that made me scared to death to fail, but one quality distinguished him from all the other doctors: I knew that for him the most important thing in all the world was saving lives, and that his scoldings, his demands, his total attention were not meant to make me feel naughty or good, but only to make me healthy. I also knew that his severity stemmed from pure love!

Choosing a medical doctor is much the same process as choosing a psychotherapist; the single most important ingredient (assuming medical credentials) is whether you like each other. Do you feel comfortable talking to the doctor and *does he listen to you?* Listening seems to be an art form that is not too common among today's physicians. Does the doctor see you as unique? Does he want to hear your hunches about yourself, your experiences and observations, before he makes any judgments? Is he willing to work with you in a flexible way, exploring many possibilities? I suspect that to some degree at least, the popularity of diet organizations reflects the dissatisfaction of many people who have given up the search for an internist who understands how they feel. Maybe they should be looking for a formerly fat doctor!

For years I assumed that I could not possibly diet in a group situation. It would be too embarrassing, and I was too shy. So I struggled along with individual psychotherapy, and with one internist at a time. It was simple desperation that made me begin to consider an alternative.

My first experiment occurred several years ago. With fear and trepidation, I went with my husband to a very fancy spa in Florida where there was a "total program," including delicious meals of 600 calories a day, exercises, massage, facials, sauna, steam—the works! On the first day I had to be fitted for a sweat suit, and the only one that fit was a man's size; I was mortified. There was also a medical examination in which the doctor called me a "bad girl." *But nothing terrible happened.* I talked back to the doctor—something I had never had the courage to do before. I said, "I'm sorry, but I will not permit you to talk to me as if I were four years old. As a matter of fact, no one ought to talk to a four-year-old that way either. I'm a woman in my fifties, and I have suffered and struggled with dieting all my life. I don't need you to make me feel guilty." He was a nice man; he looked shocked and contrite and apologized. No one had ever said that to him, and I think it gave him something to think about.

I discovered that I *loved* being taken care of by so many people—the daily massage and facial was a luxury beyond my wildest dreams. The woman who gave me a facial every day belonged to Overeaters Anonymous and one night she took me to one of their meetings. While I found the rigidity of their rituals unsuitable for me, the experience of being in another kind of group situation was not unpleasant at all. In fact, the only trouble with that fancy spa was that ten days there was enough to leave us at the brink of bankruptcy. What I learned there was that it was not a problem for me to diet in a group situation—I did not feel violated by the lack of privacy. In fact, I began to feel that group support was essential.

It was about two years later that I arrived in Durham, North Carolina. I was scared to death all over again—shy, embarrassed, wondering what in the world would happen to me. We got there three days before my medical examinations were to begin so that my husband could help me find a place to live and I could get acquainted with the town. During those three days I gained about five pounds from sheer nervousness. Every meal was the "Last Supper"! The day of the tests finally arrived and the ritual was under way—two full days of tests more complicated and extensive than anything I'd ever been through. It wasn't so bad after all. Most of the people undergoing the same procedures were just as scared and shy as I was; and many of them were a lot more overweight than I. There were also some fairly skinny people, who told us they were having their "getting-out tests," and they were enormously kind, helpful and encouraging. The staff was warm and reassuring and I felt an immediate esprit de corps among my fellow inmates. We understood each other; we had all been through the same agonies, and we had the same poignant, shimmering hopes. Maybe this time . . .

About 40 percent of the people at my motel were on the Rice Diet or one of the other diets for which Durham has become famous. What I soon discovered is that Durham is heaven for fat people! Half the people running around the town are in sweat suits, and every department store carries extra-large sizes. Nobody laughs at fat people—they're the biggest and best industry in town besides tobacco!

The advantage of our being together was that we felt genuine compassion for each other. Whatever the complaint, there was true empathy among us about being hungry, having sore feet, feeling exhausted. We all felt better because we understood each other completely.

I wrote in my journal:

> Riding on the bus to breakfast this morning was absolutely hilarious. Catherine admitted that last night she just couldn't stand it another minute—she had ordered a hamburger from room service at nine o'clock. We all went crazy! I wanted to know *every detail* about the experience. Had juice from the hamburger seeped through the roll? Was it rare, medium or well done? Did it come with potato chips? And pickles? We were all screaming with laughter at seven-thirty in the morning. Someone wanted to know the exact circumference of the hamburger. Someone wanted to know did she eat it quickly or slowly; how many times did she chew with each bite? Catherine supplied us with every mouth-watering detail. Nobody in the "outside world"

could possibly have understood why we thought all this was so excruciatingly funny.

Edith went home yesterday. A group of her closest friends bought a charm for the charm bracelet she always wears. On one side was printed what she weighed when she came, and on the other side was her going-home weight! What a nice thing to do!

I'm beginning to feel sad about leaving Durham. I thought I'd be dying to get *out*—like getting out of prison—but I miss the people who have left already, and realize how much we have meant to each other. There have been so many beautiful people who have helped me so much with such loving encouragment and understanding.

I'll never forget this place and my three and a half months here. It has been such a turning point in my life. No matter how ready one may be, compassion, concern, understanding are terribly important. One has to find them, somewhere, somehow.

When I went for tests today, there was a whole line-up of new people coming in. I see the look in their eyes—of self-disgust—and I know that in a week or two that will be gone. They will stop feeling that they are horrible because by then they will be getting to know each other, and liking each other. When you begin to care a lot about other fat people, you can begin to perceive your own beautiful qualities.

Living in Durham for three and a half months taught me that it was necessary for me to be with a group that provided encouragement and reinforcement. I also learned that I needed a flexible group relationship. Unlike Weight Watchers or Overeaters Anonymous, or some of the behavior modification groups, it was entirely up to me to choose when and for how long I wanted to be with the other people.

I spent a great deal of my time alone—taking long walks,

swimming, writing letters, resting. At other times, if I felt like it, I could have constant companionship. I ate three meals a day with the other "Ricers," but beyond that I was free to choose. It had taken me so many years of searching and experimentation to find the right setting. Fortunately, there are now so many alternatives, so many possibilities, that each of us can find our niche if we keep working for it.

The Environment

It is certainly easier and less expensive to diet at home. Some people can do it, but there are a great many others who will never lose weight and keep it off unless they completely change the environment in which they diet. It was a frightening decision for me to leave home, and I finally was influenced to do so by two sessions I had with a psychiatrist who tried to use hypnosis with me. While I did not go into a trance state, the sentences that she gave me to repeat to myself over and over again seemed to synthesize everything I had been working toward in many years of psychotherapy:

1. For my body, overeating is a poison.
2. I need my body to live.
3. I owe my body this respect and protection.

I was now fifty-four years old; I knew I was endangering my life; I wanted to live as long as I possibly could and there was no other way to work toward that goal than to be in the best possible health.

I lead a complicated and busy life; it is necessary for me to keep writing if we are going to continue to live in the style to which we have unfortunately become accustomed. I knew that if I went to Durham I would have to use a frightening amount of our financial resources. I am surrounded by people whom I love and whom I would miss. The separation from my husband was, of course, the worst part of it. My daughter is grown and on her own—which certainly made my decision a great deal easier. But I was worried about what would happen to my husband—an absent-minded professor who has high-level thoughts and brilliant perceptions, but needs to be reminded of such things as the necessity to eat and sleep and keep dental appointments and take clothes to the laundry. I admire and respect the greater equality of young marriages today, but we are old and set in our ways—and for better or worse, Larry did not know how to shop or cook or take care of household matters, or so I thought. We had learned long before to give each other plenty of breathing space—we had spent many weeks apart pursuing our own special interests—but I knew that if I went to Durham, it would be the longest time we had ever been separated, and that it would be a great hardship for both of us. The fact that he gave me total support and encouragement helped greatly, of course. I was extraordinarily lucky because his attitude was such a helpful one: "If *you* need to, do it."

Almost everybody was shocked by my decision. A few were greatly admiring because I was strong enough to fight for what I felt I needed to do. The day before I left New York, a friend told me: "As far as I am concerned, you are a beautiful woman, and I couldn't care less whether you lose weight or not. But I have to tell you that you are an inspiration to me. You make me want to try to have the courage to face my problems, to change my life."

While I was away, the outpouring of love was overwhelming: telegrams, flowers; letters from people who hated writing letters! I never felt cut off or alone; people called me constantly to keep in touch, tell me they admired me, or wish me good fortune. At one point—a low period when I hadn't lost any weight for several days—a friend called at midnight, waking me up, and said, "I just wanted to tell you I love you and you are a wonderful person," and hung up! It was just the lift I needed.

But the important thing was that while I still felt very much connected to home, family and friends, *I was away from everyone.* Nobody could ask me to do anything for him; nobody could ask me to solve his problems; I didn't have to give any lectures; and I wrote articles only when I felt like it.

I was fearful of anything that interrupted the routine. Several friends suggested that they'd like to visit me. On the phone one night, Wendy said, "I can't *wait* to see how you look! Maybe I could get off from work and visit you." I found myself retreating from such overtures. I seemed to need my isolation.

If you have tried for years and years to lose weight at home and have always failed, I think it is important, sooner or later, for you to consider total disengagement from your current life at home. I know all the rational arguments against doing this: having to get sick leave or maybe even losing a job; terrible financial strain; children and a spouse who need care. We all think we are indispensable, but the truth is that other people *can* get along without us for a few months, and that financial resources usually *can* be found if we try hard enough. And this may be shocking, but I really mean it: *Think cancer.* That is the disease that frightens us the most, so it is the most effective one to use. Just suppose you got cancer—what would happen? A way would be found for you to get the care you needed. Other people would take over your responsibilities. Money would somehow be found to do everything possible to cure you. Or let's take a less dramatic happening—a broken hip, a car accident, a mild heart attack, a slipped disk. Physical catastrophe mobilizes everyone and ways are found to meet the disaster.

Obesity is a serious disease; it is a killer. Some people simply cannot diet if relatives and friends are making demands on their time and energy; some relationships are so fraught with constant sabotage that there is no way out but to disappear until the job is done. When, in addition, very serious problems must be solved sooner or later in order to break the pattern of overeating, it is essential that there be time spent alone to think matters through before necessary decisions can be made about dramatic actions—such as getting a divorce or going back to work or changing jobs.

The greatest advantage of being away from home is that you have time to think about yourself all the time; *you are finally the most important person in your life.* This is reinforced constantly by the doctors and other personnel who are caring for you. On the Rice Diet program, the doctors are not the least bit interested in how your mother-in-law is feeling, or whether or not Johnny is doing well in reading, or if your husband has a cold or your family is living on TV dinners. The only person they are interested in is you. In the several behavior modification programs which also take place in Durham, there is much more attention paid to one's "real life" back home, and there are daily discussions which help to guide each patient to deal more effectively with his or her home problems. Dr. Kempner (the originator of the Rice Diet) says he has no patience with psychology, and unfortunately, there are no formal discussions or counseling as part of the program. But large amounts of TLC (tender, loving care) were given every day by all the doctors, nurses and technicians. When they recognized serious emotional disorders, the patient was referred to a therapist through university resources. I felt that some of the behavior modification programs, while more focused on psychological factors, were not concerned enough with medical problems and were nowhere near as thorough in terms of medical examinations and supervision. In my view, while each type of program had great assets for certain people, a combination of both approaches would have been more effective.

There are people who cannot benefit from group living or an institutional approach; it doesn't suit their personality or their stage of life or their unique circumstances. I described one such example in Durham:

Catherine is someone who ought not to be here. She is a fascinating woman. I was attracted to her the first day I got here. She's in her early seventies. She's a pediatrician. She was a pioneer in maternal and infant care and worked mostly in clinics in ghetto areas in Chicago. The stories of her life and work and travels are fascinating.

She came here at the insistence of two daughters because of high blood pressure and some overweight, although she is far from obese. She hates it here, cut off from her friends and her work. She stays here because her children and doctors tell her she might have a stroke, and she's scared, but each day she seems to become more lethargic, more forgetful. And oh, how she cheats! Most of it seems to be quite unconscious—she "forgets" the meals she orders from the restaurant. The more people try to infantilize her by protecting her, the more she rebels, like a child, and eats things she's not supposed to. She's always surprised when she doesn't lose any weight, assuring everyone she's behaving perfectly.

She should have been allowed to live—and die—with her boots on. She wants to go home and volunteer her services to a health center. She misses her friends and all the community activities that were her life blood. The longer she stays, the more she becomes convinced that she's old and sick.

No one ought to be allowed to decide what each of us needs—that's up to us!

Total Focus on Dieting

One of the reasons I found leaving home so essential was that it made it possible for my entire life to revolve around dieting, exercising and losing weight. It seems to me that when one has a great deal of weight to lose, total focus on dieting is the only possible way to do it, whether one stays at home or goes away.

After I returned from Durham, a friend of mine went there and wrote me the following letter:

Dearest Eda,

I keep writing long, long letters to you in my head. (When I'm out walking, of course.) But sitting down to write a real letter is another matter. Can you believe? I don't have the time! Not long after what we laughingly call dinner—after I've walked "home" and have soaked my poor feet in hot water with Epsom salts and have taken my nightly swim—I fall into bed like a tree crashing down in the forest and *don't move* till the next morning. And my days are busy, busy, busy, with walking and other exercise activities. I thought I would have so much free time! I feel caught up in some kind of cataclysmic time warp, as if the days down here have only sixteen hours instead of twenty-four, and there are only four days per week instead of seven. How fast it goes! I suppose it's all that coma-like sleeping that's throwing everything else out of the usual time frame.

The diet has to become an obsession, at least for a while. Maybe it takes an obsession to get rid of a compulsion! Leaving home makes this much easier, but if leaving home is truly impossible (and I think that must be questioned in all situations), then you have to plan your life at home so that it centers around your diet. It will not hurt your children or your spouse if there are no junk foods around; quite the reverse—everybody will be better off. It may mean making up one's mind that *all* restaurants are out—at least for a couple of months. Fat people tend to start salivating the minute they walk into a restaurant, and by the time they have unfolded the napkin they are starving! For some people a total focus on a diet may mean keeping very busy—going to museums, movies, plays, sporting events (no hot dogs!), parties; dancing, bowling or playing golf. For other people a total focus on dieting may mean resting a great deal, taking naps, spending a good proportion of time alone. I know one woman who hired a cook for three months so she never had to prepare food for her family. Total focus means finding the best possible ways of being kind to yourself, whatever that may involve.

It may mean buying a new dress or suit after every ten pounds; it may mean treating yourself to massages; it may mean joining a health club and sitting in a sauna. It may mean buying expensive perfume or going to a barbershop for a shave and a scalp treatment. If you are going to try to diet at home, it means sitting down with the family and telling them just how serious you are and just how much help you need. It probably means making a list of all the "chief saboteurs" in your life, and *not seeing any of them* for several months at least. That may include not going to dinner at your parents' house or the homes of your gourmet friends. It may mean staying away from annual picnics, camping trips, banquets and bridge parties.

It is necessary to focus full attention on the task at hand. Anything else is self-defeating and accounts for most of the failures. One woman told me that she found that going to a Weight Watchers class once a week was just not enough to keep her total attention on the diet, so she looked up four different groups within travel distance of her home, and went to each one, four days a week!

Total focus means making demands on other people and relinquishing a great many of the roles that we think make us indispensable. We need TLC in large doses, and we have to care enough about ourselves to demand it. It is amazing how other people can rise to the occasion when we finally scream, "Help!"

I know of no other approach to help you reach this total focus except to reiterate that if you think about what happens when one becomes seriously ill, you will know that there are ways to get the care and attention you need. If you developed a fatal or a chronic disease, what would happen? Money would be found somewhere, somehow; you would get the care you need from family, friends, and community services. You would not be left to die in some hospital room. Well, if you're fat you've *got* a fatal and a chronic disease! Adjustments can be made if you believe that. Total focus takes imagination, ingenuity and determination, and demands the cooperation of others. It can be accomplished if you really mean business.

Your Biology and the Right Diet

I have never been able to convince any doctor that different brands of aspirin affect me differently. I found one person— my dentist—who did believe that different brands of the same antibiotic affected me differently. The whole thrust of scientific research, since the discovery of the "scientific method," has been to lump us all together as if we are alike. We are not; every single person has his or her own unique physiological makeup and responses. That is the reason diets affect us differently. I once stayed on a Weight Watchers diet for two weeks and did not lose a pound. On the Atkins diet, I gained five pounds a week! On the Stillman diet, I lost weight, but very slowly. When I went to Durham, I ate nothing but fruit and rice for the first two weeks and I lost fifteen pounds. What I discovered, by sheer accident, was that salt made me hungry. I am sure this is idiosyncratic, that it doesn't apply to a great many other people, but it does to me—and the only reason I am mentioning it is so that as you try different diets, you learn to respect your own body and become highly sensitive to what is happening. *Please* don't assume this is the answer for you. What I am describing is a *method* of analyzing one's responses.

During all the years in which I was in psychotherapy, I assumed that when I went through periods of compulsive eating— when I craved sweets insanely—it was because of some emotional hangup. Of course, many periods of compulsive eating *were* related to neurotic problems and crises—but after I'd been in Durham for several weeks, I realized that something very strange had happened to me: no matter what my emotional state, I had absolutely no craving for sweets. I often dreamed of food, I often felt hungry—but always for things like chicken and salad. I thought I must be losing my mind—it was all so out of character. I had always been the kind of person who felt happiest eating a whole cake or a five-pound box of candy in one afternoon. What was happening to me? I was on the most boring diet I have ever been on in my life, and the thought of eating sweets did not appeal to me in the slightest degree.

While I am certainly not qualified to explain the medical philosophy behind Dr. Kempner's approach (I went there simply because I knew people had lost a lot of weight on the diet), one thing I came to understand very quickly: Dr. Kempner wanted to get the salt out of us. Every week we had to provide two twenty-four-hour specimens of urine. I have no idea what the units of measurement were; all I do know is that the first week my "salt count" was 670, by the second week it was 57, by the third 22, and thereafter it stayed around 11 all the time I was there. It seemed to me at first that maybe my craving for sweets had disappeared because I was eating more fruit than I'd ever eaten before, but in my gut I knew that wasn't the story—that salt was the one thing no diet had ever dealt with before and that salt made the difference.

I stayed on the diet (which eventually included certain vegetables, chicken and fish, all salt-free) for about three months. I never once craved a piece of candy. Then I had to go to Boston to give a speech that I'd contracted for a year earlier; I hadn't canceled it because it seemed to be time to test myself out in the real world. Until then, whatever cheating I'd done had only been at the motel, where there was a salt-free menu. There was to be a dinner before my speech and I had asked to have fish and vegetables without any salt. I knew as soon as I tasted the food that the chef had not complied; the food was salty, but I ate it because I was hungry and needed to rev myself up to give my speech. That night, when I got back to my hotel room, I became a wild woman, insane for some candy. There was a chocolate mint on each pillow, and I ate them immediately; then I started down to the lobby, looking for a candy machine. While I was still in the elevator, I suddenly realized that my craving for sweets was related to salt. The minute I figured it out, I was able to control myself. I went back to Durham the next day and there were no more such episodes until I went home for good. It has now happened so frequently that I know the enemy beyond all shadow of doubt: anytime I eat anything salty, I become the sugar freak I used to be. This observation appears over and over again in my journal, both during and after the period of dieting:

> Larry and I walked seven miles, round trip, to eat in a fish restaurant that we like here at the Cape. We know the owner and I felt that if I told him I couldn't have any salt at all, he would see to it that the fish was broiled with nothing on it. But the fish tasted salty to me and for the next twenty-four hours I was *starving*. I was dying for a hot fudge sundae—finally gave in and went to the ice cream parlor. But I ate only half of it and couldn't stand it—too sweet. Suddenly remembered the salty fish and realized that was when the cravings started again. Back to the un-salt mines!

> Figured I had a right to *one* lobster and *one* order of steamed clams during the *whole* summer at the Cape. A week later I sent a urine specimen to Duke: my salt count had gone back up to 212!

> Over the weekend I ate about an eighth of a pound of sliced tongue from a delicatessen. I also ate quite a bit of dried fruit, and on Monday morning I had gained three pounds! I went back on fruit and rice for two days and lost four pounds.

To lose weight and keep it off, we need to experiment until we figure out which diet is right for us. There were people in Durham who never got over their craving for sweets—obviously, salt did not affect them the way it affected me. For some people, the slightest increase in carbohydrate intake starts a whole round of overeating; the first little bit leads to more, and more leads to more—until one gives up hope all over again. Maybe some people can't tolerate dairy products, if they want to diet; maybe some can't stick to a diet unless it's all fruit and vegetables; others seem to do best with very high protein diets. I am a firm believer in the wisdom of the body—but it has to be an educated wisdom. We find our own route through trial and error and great patience. We have to sensitize ourselves to which foods seem to make us least hungry, which ones make us crave more. Our nutritional responses are just as unique as our fingerprints.

You must never ignore the necessity for balanced nutrition and medical checkups. It is also important to take vitamin and mineral supplements. I certainly don't believe in regimens of self-imposed starvation, but I believe it is possible to find a diet that feels satisfying and will meet your unique needs.

I have discovered through painful trial and error that our pattern of eating is as important as what we eat. Most nutritionists say you should eat a hearty breakfast, and insist that eating a late dinner or a bedtime snack is wrong. That kind of rigidity is just as likely to lead to failure as telling us that there is only *one perfect diet.* I found that regularity of mealtimes played a very important part in my ability to stick to the diet in Durham. Breakfast (half a grapefruit, tea, and weight and blood pressure tests!) was served from six-thirty to nine o'clock; it was best for me to get there at about seven-thirty. I can't even define what I mean by "best," except that after trying various times, I found that seven-thirty felt right. Lunch was at eleven-thirty, and that was good because it was early enough so that I didn't get too hungry. Supper was at four-thirty—which sounds disgustingly early, but when you are dieting and exercising a lot, it can feel very late in the day.

I was supposed to eat two fruits and a bowl of rice at lunch and supper. I didn't; I saved one piece of fruit from each meal, and ate one during the afternoon or saved both until bedtime. The hardest time for me to diet is in the evening, and knowing that I could have fruit before going to sleep helped to keep me from cheating.

There are probably people who can diet best if they eat a big breakfast and nothing else; there are others who are never hungry during the day, but are ravenous by 8 P.M. Some people miss breakfast most, some miss lunch most, some miss supper most. Find your own pattern; eat when it gives you greatest satisfaction and to hell with anybody's theories. Each of us has a unique biological rhythm, and the more we sensitize ourselves to it and respect it, the longer we will be able to diet.

Choosing Exercises

I love lying down; sitting is next best. If I were left to my own devices, my only exercises would be those that usually take place in bed or at the dining room table. In Durham, I finally faced the inevitable fact that no diet in the world is worth a damn unless one gives up—*forever*—being sedentary. But it is just as important to choose exercises that one can enjoy as it is to find the right diet.

In Durham, nobody offered me any choice about exercise; I was instructed to begin by walking two miles a day and eventually to work my way up to walking ten or twelve miles a day. All I remember about the first weeks of learning to walk all over again was blisters! I wrote in my journal:

Took my first walk today; about forty-five minutes. Got very tired. Tried to look and listen, experience the sun and quiet and wintry countryside. Yesterday I bought a little plant at Woolworth's and as I walked I looked for something to carry some dirt back to the motel, to put it in a bigger pot. I got absorbed in that project—found a piece of metal and a box in a pile of garbage and dug up some rich North Carolina soil! The walking was less tedious. . . .

Walked about two miles today. My feet are *killing* me. Someone recommended buying "moleskin," which I did. You line your shoes with it. I bought a wonderful pair of walking shoes, and when I break them in I know I'll be able to walk. [Tretorn—you can buy them in sporting goods stores and some shoe stores.] I also bought some Epsom salts to soak my feet in. There is a lady here who gives pedicures, and several people told me that helps a lot. I have only three Band-Aids left on my feet.

I've never been so tired, but it is physical exhaustion, not tension, and I sleep better than I've slept in years.

The pool was closed today (the energy crisis) and I really felt disappointed. I think even exercise is something you can learn to miss, if you do it regularly for a while.

The more I walked, the better I liked it. I began to be more observant of my surroundings—to really look and listen. As spring came, I would stop and look at one bud on a tree and marvel at what was about to burst forth, or I would stand and listen to a mockingbird's song for fifteen minutes.

I explored every street, every neighborhood in Durham, and by the time I came home, I knew I could walk ten to twelve miles without fainting dead away. I learned to walk so fast that now, back in New York, I never have to take buses or taxis unless the weather is really awful. In fact, it seems to me I can get places faster on my feet than in any vehicle trying to get through city traffic. Once in a while, when things are too hectic, I have to succumb to a cab or a bus, but it now feels like a deprivation. I am utterly astounded!

While I was in Durham, I stayed at a motel with an indoor heated pool (since it was winter when I arrived) and went swimming almost as regularly as I walked. I tried exercise classes, which others seemed to love, but the walking and swimming were definitely more my thing. There was one particular moment that was the turning point in my attitude toward the well-exercised body:

One of the great advantages here in Durham is Duke University; we have access to plays and concerts and lovely gardens, and some of the Ricers are even taking courses there. Last night a group of us went to a terrific concert—the Leningrad symphony was playing, with a marvelous pianist who played my favorite Rachmaninoff concerto. But something happened that interfered with my paying attention to the music. In the middle of the first piece, I suddenly looked down and realized *my legs were crossed.* My right leg was crossed over my left leg and it was hanging *down!* Swinging in the breeze, you might say! I had to use all my self-control not to shout in exultation. Only other fat people could possibly understand how I felt; when your legs and thighs are fat, you just can't do that. I haven't crossed my legs in a theater as far back as I can remember! The music was wonderful, but I was so preoccupied with my thin legs that I hardly remember it!

Until we can bring ourselves to the point of becoming truly aware of the need for body movement, we miss the opportunities that exist all around us. For example, I went to visit a friend in Los Angeles recently, and when she told me we needed to go shopping, I asked her how far the store was. She said four or five blocks, so I suggested we walk instead of drive. She looked at me as if I were some creature from Mars, and then her eyes became very thoughtful, and she grinned. The idea had never occurred to her! We had a very pleasant walk.

I have lived in the same apartment building for over eight

years, yet it never once registered that there was a health club *one block away!* Now I swim there five days a week—and resent the two days they are closed. The water is kept at a very warm temperature and I swim for pleasure, no longer because I feel I must. For others, tennis or golf or a half hour of riding an indoor bicycle—or an outdoor one where that's possible—yoga exercises or jogging may seem more pleasant.

What you have to strive for is a form of exercise that is a reward rather than a punishment. In choosing the exercise, you have to go through the same kinds of self-examination you do with the diet. Do you want to be with other people when you exercise? Do you prefer a private time to think your own thoughts? Do you want to spend a shorter amount of time in intensive exercise or take the longer amount of time needed for a walk?

Making the Decision to Begin

Some words of warning. While it is absolutely essential to experiment and make choices, some people use "shopping around" for the right diet program as a way of avoiding ever getting down to business.

There is a very fine line between interminable procrastination and patient experimentation; the important thing is to begin. There is no diet anywhere that is really *fun!* Deprivation, to one degree or another, is the name of the game. The next step is learning to endure the unavoidable discomfort without giving up the struggle.

If there is any one thing that I am sure about, it is that when this book is published, I will hear very quickly and loudly from groups of militant fat people who say that they are healthy and happy, want to remain fat, and feel they are discriminated against in a thin-oriented culture. To a degree, I understand and even agree with them.

But extreme obesity is dangerous and unhealthy; I don't see how anyone can argue that point in the face of the evidence. If nothing else, overweight is at least to some degree an indication of poor eating habits, and poor nutrition is surely hazardous to our health. What I do understand and sympathize with is the idea that we do not all need to be very thin or even moderately thin; some of us look and feel our best somewhere around "pleasingly plump"!

Once we have chosen the diet, and while we are trying to succeed at losing weight, we have to begin to get in touch with how we feel at different weights. Some of my fellow dieters in Durham simply could not stop dieting until they were quite skinny; it was the dream they had always had and nothing else made them feel good, though often they were perceived by others as being gaunt. Others found that losing perhaps half as much weight as might be considered ideal by the doctors made them feel sensationally well, and they loved the way they looked, although they were far short of skinny.

When I first returned from Durham, I had planned to lose another twenty or thirty pounds. But I discovered I felt *exactly right* after losing only fifteen additional pounds. I am still considered overweight by some doctors, but I know that if I don't respect my perception of the amount of change that is possible for me, I may blow the whole thing. Each of us has an inner image of the way we look and feel when we are at our very best, and it is in seeking for our own "natural" weight that we find a healthier weight we can live with, forever.

6

We Who
Are About
to Diet:
The Process

Choosing an individual diet is child's play compared to sticking with it! What I learned very quickly was that all kinds of new things happen to you while you are dieting. In a sense, it is like going through puberty all over again; you start out with one body and a few months or perhaps a year later, you have a totally different one. That's exactly what happens during adolescence—and we all know how crazy some teen-agers become!

While you diet, and as the weight begins to go down, every anxiety, every fantasy, every neurotic impulse, returns in full force. All during the process of dieting, it is necessary to continue to examine your feelings and behavior, to be on the alert for the self-sabotage that has always been part of the picture.

You cannot start, continue or finish a diet and keep the weight off if you still despise yourself. By the time I started to diet, I loved myself fat. I didn't love the fat, but I loved the person I had become. I hope you are now beginning to love the person you are, for that is the most essential ingredient for success.

No matter how well one has chosen a diet, dieting is never fun; it involves deprivation and discomfort, and the capacity to deal flexibly and creatively with change.

Dealing with Deprivation: Face It!

I immediately become suspicious of anyone who is cheerful while dieting strenuously! Crazy and manic some of the time, yes— but not overjoyed! One day recently I was standing in a bakery and a lady was buying a luscious chocolate cake. She commented to the saleslady, "I shouldn't buy it, but from an apple I'll never get such pleasure!" One of my earliest journal entries in Durham was:

> I have to be *insane*. I think about the glamorous, exciting, stimulating life I lead at home, and about all the wonderful foods there are everywhere, and I wonder how anyone can do what I'm doing. I'm cold and tired; my brain isn't functioning properly; I have to sleep alone in that goddamned big bed—and I'm in it, more dead than alive, by 8:30 P.M. I'm away from all the people I know—and all I have to look forward to is that maybe in a couple of weeks I'll be allowed to have some boiled, peeled, unsalted tomatoes, mushed up into a sauce on my bowl of rice, instead of fruit. Who goes to Siberia *voluntarily*??? (I did!)

I wrote endlessly about how sorry I was for myself, and I am sure that each page helped to keep me from cheating. Catharsis can be a substitute for digestion!

For those who must diet at home, the difficulties must be much greater. Having to cook tempting foods for other people and not eat them, dealing with people who try to sabotage your necessary obsession with the diet, all the normal crises that take place in any family, would test anyone's will power.

Then, there are the thin people, who cannot possibly understand our agony, no matter how much they love us. I wrote
in my journal:

> John called me last night. His insensitivity blew my mind—
> it was so uncharacteristic. He called from his office and I
> could hear voices in the background. Laughing, he said,
> "Hey, Eda, what's it like at the fat farm?" I couldn't believe
> my ears. John is a loving and tender person—was it possible
> he did not understand my reaction to that hurtful, public
> discussion of something that was so important to me? At
> first I was deeply hurt and then I got mad as hell. Got
> very depressed, couldn't sleep—got hungry, of course. Fi-
> nally, I sat down and wrote John a letter saying just how
> I felt about his talking that way—especially in front of oth-
> ers. I took a tranquilizer at 4 A.M.—the first time I've done
> that. I was so angry that I wrote John to leave me alone—
> not to call again.
>
> [A few days later] John called, terribly upset by my letter,
> so sorry and apologetic, knew he'd been insensitive, etc.
> *All I have to do is tell people how I feel!* That's what I could
> not do when I was a child—but I can now. This was a
> good experience because it reminded me that I am an adult
> now, and capable of letting people know how I feel. I also
> learned how much I care for the people who are here on
> the diet with me. I will not allow any of us to become
> the butt of jokes. These are tender, brave, hurting, compas-
> sionate, struggling people—and I love them.

I can well imagine how hard it must be to stay at home and
try to deal with one's social life, because even in Durham, among
the dieters themselves, there were almost constant inclinations
to find an excuse for a party, for a change in routine—for letting
up on the obsession. I wrote in my journal:

> I was invited to my first "farewell party." Ellen is going
> home and her closest friend invited me to a dinner she's
> organizing for Ellen. I don't approve of these parties because

I can see they are usually used as an excuse to go off the diet, but I accepted against my better judgment.

Just sitting in a restaurant is a great mistake; it made me terribly hungry. I ate too much and gained a pound overnight. Social engagements are *out* for now. I'm not ready to deal with them. I don't have to. *I can say no.*

The same pattern emerged over and over again, and each time I had to struggle with it anew:

Today I let too many people make demands on me. Arthur wanted me to walk with him to the Rice House but he walks too slowly; he's new here, and I need to go at a faster pace. Later, Jessie and Marilyn offered to drive me to the shopping center and I accepted, to be friendly, knowing I should have walked. I need to be alone more or I lose the theme of why I am here.

Even running away from home isn't a complete escape; life continues to present us with problems that look like awfully good excuses to stop dieting. I wrote:

Millie called today and is going through a terrible crisis. She's behaving very impulsively and irrationally, and I can tell it comes from some awful hurting. I'm worried half to death about her. But I will *not* let myself go to pieces and start eating. Somebody I love is *always* going to be in trouble, so I can't give in.

At another time I wrote:

David says he can't possibly diet—he's too upset because his best friend is leaving. I gave him my best professional guidance; I just said, "Bullshit!"

After being in Durham for about six weeks, I decided it was time to give myself a test; I let a friend visit me:

Liz is coming to visit me for the weekend and I'm scared to death. The only outsider who has invaded my walled fortress is Larry, and he understood my fears. Will she?

She is so loving and so excited about what I've done—but will it interfere with my routine?

Her greeting at the airport was worth whatever misgivings I had! She can't get over it. She tells me that she never really believed I could do it, but somehow she knows this is for real. Her visit is changing my schedule—we stayed up talking until midnight, so I was tired when I had to get up to leave for breakfast. I walked back and forth because I figured I wouldn't get any exercise the rest of the day. She's *lazy!* Doesn't want to walk anywhere—just sit and talk. And what harm does it do her—all 104 pounds of her!

I continued to eat all my meals except one at the Rice House. I had "Ricer chicken," baked potato and grapefruit on our one festive meal in the motel restaurant. When Liz had a chili dog in Chapel Hill, I had Sanka. It's O.K. I think I'm almost ready to make it in the outside world.

Some self-testing was inadvertent:

I slipped and fell in the bathroom last night, and really hurt my back. Am terrified that I'll begin cheating, and gain because I can't exercise. Am having a lot of pain, but took some medication so I could sleep. If I get exhausted, that weakens my resolve. Feel as if I may have broken a rib. Dr. N. told me to stay in bed with a heating pad and take Bufferin. Feel depressed, furious. It sure is hard to fight for your life! Spent day in bed but ate nothing but puffed rice and fruit. This morning I'd lost a pound. Forty-eight altogether now!

I got a taste of what it might be like to face the struggle at home, when I went to New York on my first furlough:

Home for three really pretty miserable days. Everyone I saw or spoke to on the phone was preoccupied with all kinds of problems.

In addition, the television program I came home to do was a fiasco. Larry tried hard to conceal it, but he is depressed and remote; it's an occupational hazard of creative people. He's uncertain where his work is going, doesn't know what he wants to do next, is genuinely delighted with my happiness but can't really join me in it. He's just *not there*.

I felt angry, disappointed, frustrated, lonely, and finally depressed, but I didn't start eating! R. called after the television program and said I shouldn't lose any more weight—my face is too thin. She weighs 115 pounds! It rained the whole three days. Met J. for lunch, and could see that he felt uneasy with me. When I am having my own troubles figuring out who I am, it is very frightening when an old friend treats me like a stranger. When I went to see my dentist, he hugged me and said, "You're disappearing!" Another reinforcement of my own irrational fantasies! To hell with going home!

When I got back I discovered that everyone had watched the television program at the Rice House, and their pride and excitement made me feel wonderful. It's crazy, but here, among people I've known for such a short time, I feel more at ease than with the friends and relatives at home whom I've known all my life!

Whether one diets at home or away from home, it now seems to me that having a special group to relate to, people who really understand what you are going through, is a tremendous help.

Fighting Old Patterns

Hard as it is to deal with pressures from the outside world, the pressures from within are even greater. The process of dieting itself seems to reinvoke old terrors, and feelings of guilt and depression. There is, first of all, enormous guilt about neglecting other people, if you have run away from home. We seem to develop more guilt feelings than anything else while we are growing up. If some educator could figure out just how guilt is taught and apply the same procedures to reading and writing, we'd have a nation of highly literate people!

Dieters with young children feel guilty if they keep all sweets out of the house; they feel guilty if they give such things to their children when they know they shouldn't. They feel guilty about not wanting to go to parties a spouse wants to attend. They feel guilty, most of all, simply because they are paying attention to themselves. Here is one of the many places where a daily journal is very important. I found that writing down all the things I felt guilty about helped to reveal their natural absurdity!

Fighting old patterns can, in itself, become excessive. I wrote in my journal:

> Walked about ten miles today and almost killed myself. Never have been so tired in my life—and of course am terribly hungry now. It is so hard to find a balance between doing and overdoing.

Here again, recording daily events can give you perspective and help you become flexible enough to make necessary adaptions.

One of the most important exercises while one diets is assessing when one has had enough to eat. It takes a great deal of concentration and awareness, because we are accustomed to simply eating until all the food is gone. It is also difficult not to allow food to continue to be the focus of so much of our attention. I wrote in my journal:

> There was some sort of celebration at lunch today. Apparently, a man has come back for his twenty-first annual checkup. He'd had a very severe heart attack, came here and lost a hundred pounds, and comes back for a checkup once a year. I couldn't believe it when I heard he was seventy— he looks about fifty. At any rate, his arrival is celebrated each year by a special meal—*potato pancakes* made with rice!

It's hard to believe, but they were sensational! The excitement was incredible. The noise level must have been ten times what it ordinarily is. Such glee! We behaved like little children who have been rewarded for good behavior.

There was no shortage of observations about gluttony!

There was great hilarity at the movies the other night. A man spilled his buttered popcorn on the floor and the three of us were ready to get down on all fours and eat it! We had bananas and some puffed rice with us, but it didn't help in the least. The smell of the popcorn made it impossible for us to pay much attention to the movie. We acted like giddy schoolgirls, giggling and being shushed by everyone around us.

Lester had us spellbound at lunch today, describing his cheating spree yesterday. He was in a foul mood and just couldn't stand it another minute. He went to McDonald's and bought a cheeseburger, two Big Macs, french fries and an apple fritter. Then he stopped at some other place and bought a quart of chocolate swirl ice cream—and a Tab! He was too ashamed to walk into his motel with all this junk, so he bought a shopping bag to hide it in! He's on the first floor of his motel and he didn't want anyone looking in while he gorged himself, so he closed the drapes. By now, all of us at the table had shared every mouthful! We became more and more involved and hilarious. When things quieted down, I asked him how he had enjoyed it. "You all enjoyed it more than I did," he said. "You enjoyed it vicariously—I'm the one who gained two pounds."

Talking about food helped a great deal. It was, I guess, our main topic of conversation every day—what we missed the most, what we liked the best, our favorite recipes, the first meal we would eat when we had reached our goal. The reason talking helped was that we were admitting our gluttony to each other

and finding it funny and sad rather than hateful. In ourselves
we found it disgusting—but when we recognized it in all the
others, it became a human failing for which we could begin
to feel compassion and understanding.

There wasn't one person who did not have a rationalization
for eating at least one thing more than was on the diet. For
some, it was morning coffee with cream—they said they just
could not live without it. For one, it was keeping crackers in
the room, supposedly in case an ulcer acted up again. For another, it was extra fruits, or she said she would faint. I began
keeping a green pepper and some lettuce in my room; in case
I wanted to cheat, this would be better for me than room service.
One way to stay on a diet is to choose a relatively innocuous
form of cheating as a necessary bulwark against the suffering
which leads to breaking the diet. We used to be ingenious about
finding excuses to eat; now we could turn all that ingenuity
toward making ourselves as comfortable as possible while still
dieting. I wrote in my journal:

> When you are *ready* to do something, you *can* do it. Every
> time I traveled or had to eat out or went on a picnic, I
> always made excuses for eating the wrong foods—after all,
> what could you take on a picnic except sandwiches and
> potato chips! Well, we just had a picnic. Jessie has a kitchen,
> and I wanted to begin to practice cooking before going
> home. I baked some chicken breasts and prepared "capo-
> nato"—made of onions, green pepper, tomatoes and
> eggplant. It's very simple to make, and delicious cold. We
> took it in a jar and spread it on unsalted rice wafers. I
> also made some potato salad, with vinegar and a tiny bit
> of safflower oil. It's one of the first picnics I've ever been
> on where I didn't gain weight. We went to a nearby lake
> and found picnic tables. Jessie said, "If this is dieting, it
> certainly isn't suffering!"
>
> I am learning that suffering is a form of sabotage. If one
> lets one's life become miserable, then one rationalizes that

one cannot endure it and there's an excuse to break the diet. If I'm not suffering, there is no reason to stop dieting.

After a while, even more serious forms of adversity can be met without starting to eat again:

> Coming back here from my first trip home, the airline lost my baggage. It was transferred to the wrong flight from Washington to Durham. I had a fit. All my notebooks, all my smaller-size clothes, were in that bag. The agent told me to go to the motel and call the next morning—they would put a tracer on it. I was terribly upset about it. But the next morning, in addition to having my bag returned, something else wonderful happened: I realized that last night's anger and unhappiness had not led to an eating binge; in fact, the idea hadn't even occurred to me! The secondary gains of losing have set in; I like being noticed and complimented.

On another occasion, I wrote:

> I went out yesterday morning, leaving the window open. The table with my journal on it was right next to the window, and it poured all afternoon. When I finally came in, the notebook was soaked and the writing all blurred. I howled in pain. My precious notes—how could I write a book without them?
>
> I typed out sheets as fast as I could, trying to decipher what was left of the writing, but the loss of some whole pages of notes depressed me terribly. I was so damned *mad* at myself for being so careless.
>
> [The next day] This morning it occurs to me that even though I was so upset last night, *I didn't start eating!* How amazing! I had the perfect excuse to rationalize myself into misery-needs-a-hamburger-and-a-milk-shake. But I didn't. Walking home from breakfast, I felt so triumphant.

My respect for human ingenuity increased tremendously in Durham. What lengths we would go to fool ourselves! There were a thousand rationalizations for self-sabotage. I wrote in my journal:

> We all have such wonderful excuses. One man says that every time he has to go to visit his aged mother in a nursing home, it is so upsetting that he eats all the way there and back, stopping at McDonald's and Carvel's and arriving home bilious and full of self-hatred. Another man blames his wife. He says, "She's a sensational cook; it hurts her feelings if I don't stuff myself." Another man tells me: "It's the loneliness. Ever since my wife died, I sit around every night watching television and gorging myself on junk. What other comfort is there, so easily available?"

Another trap is to stay on the diet but to eat larger quantities of the allowed foods:

> [On a visit home] I haven't cheated at all, in the sense of eating foods I'm not allowed—but I guess the quantity is what is creeping up on me, because I haven't lost any more weight. That scares me. I must be as conscious of quantity as of quality. I had better go back on rice and fruit for a while. I'm not getting as much exercise either. I am rushing all day and don't seem to have time to walk. I must find time.

> [Back in Durham] People who are still frightened of getting thin develop the most ingenious games. Carol is "starving" herself on two small salads a day. There is, however, this small detail: She is smothering the salads in Roquefort dressing, toast and bacon bits, pickled beets and corn relish!

Dealing with Fantasies

Since most of our feelings about food and fat originated in childhood, we tend to have a lot of irrational fantasies while dieting. I was shocked by my first fantasy:

I'm terribly depressed and I'm having a hard time figuring out why. I haven't lost any weight for a few days, but my God, I've been doing so well all along—what do I want? Ah—I know exactly what I want! I guess I had a fantasy that once I dieted, the weight would just disappear overnight. Instead, it's hard work. No wonder we all get discouraged; inside each one of us is probably a little child whispering, "I'm being so good, so why don't I get rewarded *this minute?*" When we were children and did something we were told to do, it is more than likely that we were given some immediate reward—even if just a kiss or a hug. I guess I still feel that if I am behaving like a good child I should get an immediate reward. Well, I *have* been rewarded. It just isn't all at once.

We have hilarious conversations about the "Eat, darling" syndrome of childhood, and what the diseases were with which we were threatened. Bobbie said her mother made her think she'd be retarded if she didn't eat: "You won't be able to read or write unless you eat all your potatoes." A real biggy is that we would disappear if we didn't eat: "If you don't eat, you'll waste away to nothing." Or: "You'll be so tiny we won't be able to see you."

One reason so many people stuck to the diet in Durham was probably that Dr. Kempner threatened us with all the horrible diseases from which we might die if we did not *diet*—an exact reverse of our childhood experiences.

This subtle reversal was evidenced by our preoccupation with our medical reports. I had always led an active life, and I rarely felt sick, although I was aware of the damage overeating was doing and knew I was a borderline diabetic. Still, I did not feel really sick, and neither did many others. One of the first things I was warned about when I arrived was that my initial health report would advise me that I was at death's door. We all got reports that made us feel it would be wise to start making arrangments with a friendly mortician. There was a lot of black humor about these reports:

> One woman said, "When my husband sees this report, he's going to want to take out three more life insurance policies on me." Sylvia warned me, "Don't get frightened—it will look like a coroner's report!" As each new group comes in, the old-timers warn them not to die of terror because they are told they are dying of fat! I guess the funniest comment was from the woman who said, "Looking at this report makes me feel very lucky I don't have syphilis; it's the only disease that isn't mentioned!"

Underneath all the joking I began to sense the fact that most of us were shifting from the child inside us who was saying we would die if we didn't eat, to the point of view of the doctors, who were telling us we would die if we did eat.

Second Puberty

During the dieting process—especially if we have chosen a diet in which we lose weight rapidly—the bodily changes make us feel very much the way a youngster feels as she moves from childhood toward adulthood. There is nothing like a rigid and strenuous diet to help one remember how shocking and disconcerting it is to be a child and for breasts to start swelling, or for one's legs to suddenly grow four inches. The physical changes are just as surprising and confusing as the emotional ones. I wrote in my Durham journal:

> I can't understand what is happening to me—I'm freezing all the time! I've lost eighteen pounds in fifteen days! I guess my poor body doesn't know what hit it. But it is very frightening; I've always been too hot, and so feeling cold all the time makes me imagine I am someone else, not myself. That scares me.

This change in body temperature has remained. It took a lot of getting used to. When I was heavy, I wore light clothes summer and winter; sweaters or wool dresses made me perspire in steam-heated rooms. Unless I slept under a light blanket, I was too hot. As I began to accumulate a new wardrobe, I had to adapt to the fact that my insulation system had been drastically and permanently revised. I wrote about other changes:

> Losing weight this rapidly causes all kinds of new sensory feelings. Even though I'm getting thinner, I feel clumsier. My feet walk faster than the rest of me knows how to keep up with! If I sit down on a hard chair too suddenly, it hurts my spine—now there's a bone sticking out at the bottom of me! I feel unbalanced and disorganized. My body is a stranger I never met before.

These feelings continue all during the period of dieting, and the more we become aware of them, the less shocked we will be by the new self-image we must deal with when the dieting is over.

The Giving of Gifts

I don't think anything turned out to be more important while I dieted than learning to give myself gifts other than food, to comfort and reward myself. It started quite unconsciously, but I learned to devote a great deal of attention to this matter as time went on:

> Walking home from breakfast, I felt discouraged and sorry for myself. No weight loss for two days, and it is such a struggle after the first few dramatic weeks. Stopped at a drugstore and bought myself an assortment of makeup that I certainly don't need. Felt like an idiot—and then suddenly realized that I had made a sensational shift in a living pattern. Ordinarily, feeling discouraged or depressed would

have driven me into a bakery or to a candy counter. I seem to have shifted to a much more sensible solution. Good for me! I was giving myself solace—but not food.

I had promised myself two chili dogs when I lost forty pounds. Instead, I bought a pair of slacks and two blouses—three sizes smaller!

Today I bought myself some perfume and sugarless bubble gum! It was either that or a Milky Way!

Had a pedicure—second time in my life. It was wonderful—so luxurious! My feet feel so much better. It was one of the many ways I must learn to give myself gifts that are not food. I've decided to have a massage once a week. Bodily pleasure without calories!

Tremendous sense of fatigue. I need to learn to pace my walking. I took a taxi back from the shopping mall instead of trying to force myself to walk both ways. I planned to swim tonight, but am accepting the fact that I am just too tired. Am consciously working at not feeling guilty about my limitations, but to admire and love what I *am* capable of doing.

Yesterday my editor called—one of my children's books sold to a paperback company for a sizable advance. I was so relieved—it will help pay for all these expenses. Today Sylvia took me with her to a cut-rate store that sells everything imaginable. I bought myself a ring for *seventy dollars!* All my rings are too big for me, and until I get home and have them made smaller, I have no rings I can wear. It was a great extravagance, and for a while this afternoon I must have been feeling guilty about it, because I got terribly hungry. I was terrified that I would order a hamburger from room service, so I went out and bought a green pepper and a banana. Then Larry called and told me he thought it was wonderful that I had bought myself a present. I suddenly felt very proud of myself. Another hurdle taken; *I can celebrate without eating!*

[After returning home] I just planted a yellow rosebush, which I'm calling my Ice Cream Rose. This morning I tore up about fifty pages of writing that just wasn't any good—almost a week's work. I was very depressed and developed an absolutely overwhelming desire for ice cream. In this part of Cape Cod there are no less than three ice cream parlors where they make their own ice cream and sauce. Ecstasy! I got in the car, my salivary glands already in full action, visions of maple nut ice cream with homemade mocha fudge sauce on top dancing in my head. As I got near the ice cream parlor, I passed a nursery and saw a sign announcing that rosebushes were on sale. I stopped to buy one and without thinking about it, I came home and planted it. It took me three hours to remember why I had started my trip, but by that time the crisis was over; I was in love with my rosebush.

One of the most important gifts we can give ourselves is clothes in smaller sizes as we lose—but we have to be careful that we don't get them too tight; that's again discouraging. I didn't buy anything in a new size until it would be loose enough to be worn with no girdle! Comfort is as important as being attractive during a period of deprivation.

Most of us tend to be the kind of people who always give things to other people, but find it very difficult to receive. It is time to do something about that while dieting. We need to let the people who care about us know how much their encouragement means to us.

Edith sends me funny clippings to amuse me, Maria sent a drawing made with rice kernels pasted on paper! I feel so cherished, so encouraged. My cup runneth over—which is a funny thing to say on a starvation diet! Last night Ted called me and made me laugh and this morning there was a beautiful letter from Larry about missing me and feeling proud of me. It makes such a difference; they feed my soul—which is very nice when I'm starving my body!

I tell people how much their letters and phone calls mean to me. Last night Paul called to sympathize with my struggle. He calls Dr. Kempner "that Nazi who is starving you to death!" I protest that he is the "good German" who wants me to live—but I enjoy the game of being sorry for myself. Larry called and told me not to push myself too hard on the walking. It's wonderful to get so much approval. I'm very lucky; I'm trying to encourage some of the others to let their families know they need support and understanding, not scoldings.

Another kind of gift is to change your routine when you get restless and unhappy:

I went to Duke University yesterday and bought a whole bunch of tickets for myself, Margaret, Catherine, Kay and Sylvia. We are going to two dance recitals, one lecture, one opera and two concerts in the next six weeks! Getting dressed up and going out is not a luxury, it's a necessity.

I think probably the best words ever said on this subject were by Will Stanton, writing in *Reader's Digest:* "People who want to lose weight, the diet writers say sternly, must adopt a no-nonsense attitude. Hogwash. If we're going to diet, we need all the nonsense we can get. All the soft lights and music and sweet talk and dancing and trips to the racetrack and shopping sprees and everything else that's fun and calorie-free."

As a rule, fat people are not at all talented in the fine art of self-forgiveness. We might never have become fat if we had that ability. We have tended to understand everyone else's imperfections, but are intolerant of our own:

I think Betty is going to make it. Last night she really went on a wild spree—steak dinner, wine, strawberry shortcake for dessert! She doesn't seem to hate herself for this fall from grace. She laughed *lovingly* at her own human fallibility. She knows we will all fail once in a while. She's not mad at herself today. She said, "Listen, girls—where does it say I have to be perfect?"

Ordered "Ricer fried chicken" from room service and ate it almost in one gulp. Felt sick and furious at myself. But I know what I have to do. *I have to forgive myself,* or it won't stop. I am not a perfect human being, and I haven't cheated much at all. Everybody has a breaking point and I reached mine. Forgive! Forgive!

Inevitably one does things that seem quite crazy—but they only seem so if we don't understand what they mean. When I got home I proceeded to give away every piece of clothing I owned—probably about two thousand dollars' worth of dresses and coats. I regret this craziness terribly now—but I am not angry at myself. It was a dumb thing to have done, because by the time I went to Durham, I was buying very beautiful materials and having my dresses made for me. Many of them could have been redesigned; I miss some of those beautiful clothes.

The worst of my insanities was this: When my mother died, I inherited her mink coat—a true luxury that I loved. When I came home from Durham, it was slightly big for me—but it was luxurious and the overlapping kept me extra warm. Although there was really no necessity to do anything to it, I spent $350 having it made smaller. That ruined it; now there is no overlap and I freeze to death in it. I destroyed something beautiful and precious to me. At first I was furious and grief-stricken at my craziness. Then one night, a friend came for dinner and I told him the whole story about the coat. He said: "I don't know why—or what the connection is—but that story reminds me of something that happened to me when I was a kid. I had an older cousin whose family was much richer than mine. I was given all his hand-me-downs and I hated it. One coat was impossible, it was so big, but my father kept insisting, 'You'll grow into it.' ''

You'll grow into it. When Paul said that I knew instantly why I had behaved in such an idiotic fashion. I was afraid that if I kept any of my clothes or didn't make the coat smaller, I might gain the weight back and grow into them. As soon as I understood the unconscious motivation, I could forgive myself. Sometimes, though, we have to forgive ourselves even if we can't understand something we do. Dieting strenuously is enough of an explanation for going a little crazy.

The Terror of Being Thin—As the Reality Approaches

As we are forced to perceive that we are no longer obese, all the old terrors reassert themselves. I wrote in my journal:

> The other day Sylvia said, "With every ten pounds I lose, I feel more and more like a forty-seven-year-old Lolita!" Agnes nodded and added, "I don't know if it is simply because I have more energy and vitality or whether I have become less ashamed of my body—but whatever it is, I seem to have more sexual feelings than I ever had in adolescence."
>
> I'm sure that some of the people who quit and go home have been frightened by such feelings. Others seem to lie back and enjoy it! There is every opportunity for finding new sex partners when one lives in motels! For many, this is the first experience in really "breaking loose" and the reactions are what one would expect, ranging from guilt and fear to a lusty exultancy. We have had a few conversations about masturbation and I am appalled by the number of middle-aged women who do not allow themselves this pleasurable activity.
>
> At the clinic the other day there was a woman I'd never

seen before—very loud and funny—who, after asking a lot of questions about what life is like here, said, "I'd sure like to have the vibrator concession down here!" What many of us do talk about is the pleasure of having massages while one is dieting. That is one of the busiest industries here—and a relaxing and sensual comfort for many. There is a lot of panic, often concealed by bravado. A few days ago a woman in the lobby said, "Well, what shall I do tonight? Cheat on the diet or cheat on my hubby?"

Helen has stopped exercising. She gained ten pounds during one week at home. She is totally focused on food and feelings of deprivation. She "Oh"s and "Ah"s over every candy store and ice cream parlor we pass, suffering loudly. She wants to talk about food while I want to talk about clothes. I finally confronted her with the self-sabotage that is going on. She says she knows she is afraid of becoming thin, but doesn't know why. We talked for hours and figured out part of it anyway. She was married to such a bastard that she feels sure she is unable to judge men at all; if she gets thin, if men are attracted to her, might she make another terrible mistake in judgment? "Better stay fat and avoid all that misery," she says bitterly.

Jerry says he really means business; no matter what, he is going to stay here until his weight is normal and his diabetes arrested. He has a very limited amount of money and he squanders it; he doesn't exercise enough and he eats about five times as much fruit as he's supposed to be having. He is unaware of the self-sabotage that's going on. When he leaves here he has to find a new job and an apartment, and deal with the fact that he is now divorced. He seems quite unaware of the ways in which he prolongs his stay here, to avoid dealing with going home.

Chris was one of the best dieters here. She never cheated, she walked a lot, she even jumped rope in the motel hallway!

This past week or so I've begun to realize that she's eating in the motel restaurant and spending a great deal of time with the people who are "the cheaters." I found out from one of her friends that she had been told three weeks ago that she was well enough to go home. Chris has been here eight months. Before she left home, her husband told her he wanted a divorce to marry someone else—probably the reason she got so heavy. She's made him wait all this time, hoping he'd change his mind, but he hasn't. She doesn't want to go home and face it all.

Annie has been ready to go home for weeks, but she stays on, playing tennis, flirting, saying she wants to lose "just another couple of pounds." Her children came to visit her for their spring vacation, and she looked harassed, aggravated and frustrated. She told me, "I'm not going home until the very last second I have to!" She hopes her husband will put up with her absence until school closes for the summer. While the children are in school, he can manage with a housekeeper.

Maybe there will be fewer fat people, now that women feel freer to decide not to get married and have children. I said this to Annie and her eyes filled with tears. I'd hit a nerve, I guess. I have a feeling she's on the verge of telling me what she wishes she had done with her life. I hope I can convince her it's all still possible; maybe she can go home and get started!

There's one woman here who can't bear to go home because all her children are grown up. She began to gain a great deal of weight during her youngest child's last year in high school. She told me, "I raised my children to be independent. I did a wonderful job. But I forgot all about preparing *me!* I always wanted to be good to everyone— make them happy. You want pie—I'll bake pie; you want rice pudding—I'll make rice pudding. Now I have to learn to be good to myself. I forgot *me*, because that's harder than all the rest."

A woman returned just the other day. She had been here for four months, had lost seventy pounds, went home, stayed for about three months, gained forty pounds back, and here she is again. In the pool this morning we had the following conversation:

JANE: I just can't do it at home. All day long the kids are eating potato chips, peanuts, ice cream—and I have to cook big meals for my husband, and there are always people dropping in, so I bake a lot of cookies and cakes. . . .

ME: All that stuff isn't really good for them either.

JANE: I know. (Laughs) In fact, my daughter told me, "Mom, we want you to stay home. Please. We'll give up all that junk, we won't have any of it in the house, we'll all go on your diet, if you'll just stay home."

ME: So? That's a pretty good offer.

JANE: I guess I really like it better here!

Unless she gets around to examining why she is happier here, and what she can do about it, I suppose this pattern will go on indefinitely.

What we all have to figure out, sooner or later, is how to deal with our reality in a responsible way and yet leave ourselves enough room to live satisfying, fulfilling lives. It is so easy to blame everyone else for our failures. My most popular rationalization is that at home I have to eat in too many restaurants because I travel a lot and have so many social and business activities. It's going to be like that for the rest of my life. I will have to find some way to deal with my reality. I will have to cook and eat at home more of the time and find some way to go to restaurants without eating foods I can't have. I have to make the decision and do the planning. It's my free choice.

I wrote in my journal:

> Larry is going to a meeting in Paris and Phyllis asked
> if I was going along. I said, "Why should I go to Paris
> when I can't eat?" She smiled and said, "Paris is also where
> the best designers' clothes happen to be!" It had never occur-
> red to me! It is also, for me, the most beautiful city I have
> ever seen. It shocks me to realize that my immediate re-
> sponse had to do with food, when there is so much to feed
> my soul there. My God, but it is so hard to change one's
> orientation to life!

Gluttony can be replaced by vanity; senses of sight and smell
and touch can be developed to new intensities, as taste is relin-
quished:

> We took Bev and Wendy for ice cream and I had iced tea.
> It seemed very simple; I would rather have my Halston
> pants suit, size 12, than ice cream!
>
> I realized recently how differently I *look* at things than I
> did a year or two ago. I was at a Monet exhibit at the Metro-
> politan Museum of Art, and was so profoundly moved. I
> walked more slowly, looked more deeply. I finally said, "It's
> such a feast, it hurts my eyes"—and then realized the word
> I'd used. There are other ways to "feast" besides eating.

After my first visit home to New York, I wrote:

> I had a wonderful time. Everybody gasping with delight!
> I stopped over in Washington on the way home, having
> arranged to meet a friend in the airport, who was on his
> way somewhere else. He pretended not to recognize me
> and walked right by, then did a clownish double take. I
> *loved* it! Later I was waiting at a corner for a cab. The
> driver said, "It's always a pleasure to pick up a pretty lady!"
> I looked around to see whom he was talking about; he meant
> *me!*

What seems strange to me now is that the above was written
in my journal when I had lost only thirty pounds—less than

half of what I was ultimately to lose. But I *felt* marvelous; I was far from sylphlike, but I was thinking of myself as being attractive and that made all the difference.

We begin to change our own priorities—partly because we like ourselves better, and partly because inevitably we find ourselves influenced by the attitudes of other people. The degree to which we become increasingly selective about which reactions to accept or reject is the degree to which we are likely to succeed or fail.

7

The World
Is So Full
of French
Pastries

We live in a totally schizophrenic society which assures us on the one hand that skinny is beautiful, healthy, necessary—and on the other hand presents us with an environment in which we are constantly bombarded by every imaginable temptation to eat.

Soon after I had returned from Durham, my husband and I went to Provincetown for a day's outing. We were spending a few days at our summer home on Cape Cod—the first vacation together after the long separation. We felt festive, relaxed; it was time to have fun together.

Approaching Provincetown, we stopped for a while to walk along the magnificent dunes, to take in all the breath-taking scenery available to us that was noncaloric. So far, so good. But then we headed into the central part of the town and I began to realize that for the rest of my life there would be one part of vacationing that was going to drive me nuts. Within one block, we were assailed by the signs and smells of fried clams, Portuguese soup, hot dogs, fresh bread and pastry, home-made ice cream, pizza and, God help us, a chocolate factory!

Since we have always indulged ourselves on vacations, I suddenly realized how much self-denial the day was going to involve; I wouldn't have any more fun. I felt deprived and depressed.

The task each of us faces is to continue to struggle against old patterns and to face the inevitability of a society that will entice us, try to seduce us into eating, everywhere we turn. I had to begin to try to figure out how I could still feel I was on vacation without food being a central focus of attention.

One of the kinds of vacation that my husband and I have always enjoyed the most is a cruise. It is the one vacation where no one can call you on the telephone or ask you to do anything, so it represents a total escape from our usual responsibilities. About six months after I returned from Durham, we took a two-week cruise. At first I thought it was one of my more stupid decisions. I had placed myself in an environment where the eating of food in association with being on a vacation reaches some sort of pinnacle. That luxury ship was a microcosm of the United States, where overeating has reached proportions that border on obscenity.

One day the ship had an outdoor "picnic lunch," an informal buffet near the pool. I wrote down what was being served. Here is the list:

Tossed salad, watermelon, fresh fruits, cheese and crackers, thirteen different kinds of cake (including almond torte, rum babka, cheese cake, meringues with sauce, and French pastry), strawberries and cream, cranberry sauce, roast beef, turkey, corned beef, tongue, cold chicken, ham, pork, applesauce, pickles, olives, relishes, tomatoes, curried rice, cheese and ham salad, chicken salad, potato salad, hard-boiled eggs, fried rice balls, fried fish sticks, potato pancakes, fried raisin dumplings, pizza, fried apple fritters, crabmeat croquettes, spareribs, meatballs in tomato sauce, manicotti, beef stew, hamburgers, hot dogs, rolls and butter, and chicken cacciatore.

This was just lunch. The breakfast menu offered at least thirty different dishes. At every dinner we were offered about ten appetizers, five soups, several kinds of pasta, about ten main dishes and five desserts. At midnight every night, there was a complete buffet dinner. If you were hungry between meals, there was a small restaurant where you could get free pizzas. For those who were still feeling malnourished, there was twenty-four-hour room service, as well as consommé served at 11:30 A.M. and tea with pastry at 4 P.M.

I gained only three pounds in fourteen days! A miracle of self-control! At first I was sure the cruise would be a total disaster, that I would gain back everything I'd lost and be fat again; I was terrified. But much to my surprise, I discovered that my increased self-awareness was sensitizing me to the temptations in the world around me and that I was beginning to be able to say a resounding *no* to this kind of revolting gluttony. It turned out to be a good experience after all, because I found myself feeling as if I were on a vacation without uncontrolled eating.

I don't think I will ever be able to eat in restaurants or go on vacations without getting into some trouble. It is simply more than most of us can handle, no matter how profoundly we have made the choice not to be fat. I think we have to deal forthrightly with the fact that we cannot handle all temptation, that will power has its limits. What this means for me is eating in restaurants as little as is humanly possible, thinking carefully about vacations that will feed my *soul*, and losing enough weight so that I will always have about ten pounds leeway for periods of total relaxation for a few days, followed by a period of stringent dieting. Maybe there are fat people in this world who really and truly train themselves to eat only what is good for them, and who develop a dietary program that they can stick to for the rest of their lives without feeling deprived. I would like to meet one of them; I never have. I am sure that a diet of salad, vegetables, chicken, fish and fruit would seem magnificent to me on a desert island. As long as I live in the United States and as long as I am not blind and don't lose my sense of smell, I am going to feel deprived every time I pass a Pizza Hut or Fried Clam Bar. And since there is hardly a day in my life when I do not pass at least fifty restaurants and at least ten bakeries, what I must continually do is to try to recognize my cravings and deal with them at least 90 percent of the time, allowing myself a 10 percent failure quotient, saved for vacations or party time.

One of the clearest examples of the double messages with which we are constantly bombarded is found in the women's magazines. There is at least one diet program recommended in every issue, accompanied by an article that tells us we are killing ourselves with overeating and that this particular diet is foolproof if we stick to it. That may take up perhaps five pages throughout the magazine, including recipes. At the same time, there will be at least fifty pages (a conservative estimate) of full-page color pictures of all the kinds of foods that are presumably going to kill us off.

There is nothing we can do except show as much control as we can and forgive ourselves for the fact that sometimes we fail. We need to celebrate our victories and not dwell on our failures. After returning home from Durham, I wrote in my journal:

> Yesterday I took a half hour walk in the neighborhood. I passed about ten Italian restaurants, fifteen Chinese, five Spanish, two French, a pancake place, a bagel place, four Jewish delicatessens, about fifteen bakeries, a Greek restaurant, and four ice cream parlors. Also Zabar's [a gourmet

center—one of the most famous places for gluttons in all
the world]. And this was on a quiet Sunday morning!! My
salivary glands were in a state of total agitation. I stopped
and bought a banana and ate it *very slowly*.

Second-Class Citizenship

A major environmental influence on us is the fact that in our
culture even "pleasingly plump" is somehow considered "lower
class." Fat people are treated quite differently from thin people,
and that inevitably affects our struggle. We continue to identify
with fat people and are suddenly much more aware of subtle
nuances in people's attitudes. For example, I wrote in my Durham journal:

> This morning Dr. G. said, "Haven't you noticed? Fat people
> always look stupid and lower class." She said it very casually,
> while I was having my blood pressure checked. I was terri-
> bly shocked. I went back to my room and looked at my
> "before" pictures (I've seen lots of other people's pictures
> too) and there is a germ of truth in this—but it's an attitude.
> I think of myself as an animated, intelligent-looking person,
> but in the picture I *do* look stupid! I think the camera catches
> something we feel about ourselves; we are caught off guard,
> and a strange kind of body language takes over.

Another time I wrote:

> Fat people *are* second-class citizens! I'm just beginning to
> realize what a protected life I've led. I never noticed any
> slights from strangers; if there were any, I guess it never
> mattered—the people who loved me loved me, and that was
> all that mattered. Now salespeople are more gracious, men
> offer to be helpful, hold doors open, offer to carry suitcases,
> hold the elevator door, start conversations with me in the
> motel lobby—are far more attentive. It infuriates me that
> forty pounds could make such a difference.

While I was home, a woman in the elevator said, "Boy, did you lose weight!" I said, "Thank you." And then I was shocked by my saying that. The unconscious agenda was perfectly clear; if someone tells you you've lost weight, it's a compliment—like getting smart or rich. Why should I thank somebody for telling me I lost weight?

My favorite story in this connection—I call it "The Fat One Strikes Back!"—is recounted in my journal:

Maxine is back here for her final medical checkup. She lives in a wealthy suburb of Cleveland. All her friends go to one particular saleslady in the dress department of a very fashionable store for their clothes. Maxine wore a size 20 and this dress department only had dresses up to size 16. But those were the best clothes in town, and she used to go in to talk to the saleslady about the possibility of her choosing a particular dress and then perhaps ordering it in a larger size. The saleslady would give her a withering look and assure her that "these styles" never, never come in larger sizes. She would assure Maxine that very few "really nice things" come in large sizes. "You would do much better going to the ready-to-wear women's department of another, cheaper store," she would advise, in a patronizing tone of voice. Maxine was furious but always behaved in a polite and obsequious manner in these confrontations. Then Maxine came to the Rice House and lost eighty pounds. She now weighs 110 pounds and wears a size 6.

Back in Cleveland, she went to the saleslady, who did not recognize her but waited on her with great courtesy and patience. Maxine tried on every single dress in her size. She kept each one on for fifteen minutes, undecided about how she felt about it. She turned down dress after dress, with such comments as, "This looks cheap," or "This is sleazy material," or "This is cut very badly." All during this two-hour session, the saleslady never lost her cool. She chatted on and on—polite, friendly, attentive. At the end of her performance, Maxine said, "Now I want to tell you who I am. I've been here many times before. My name is Mrs. Gardner. When I was heavy, you always treated me with contempt. You were rude and unkind. I will never buy a dress in this store and I am going to tell the manager why!" When she told us this story at lunch, we all applauded. It was, I suppose, a childish revenge, but necessary.

When I was fat I was under the impression that people treated me with respect. Once I had lost a great deal of weight, I began to suspect that maybe the reason I never noticed any slights was that *I* had behaved differently. When I was back home, I wrote in my journal:

> I walked into the corner grocery market. The owner said, "Hello, skinny lady, how are you?" I felt annoyed by this continuing discussion of my size and answered curtly, "I'm fine," and started down an aisle. He called after me, "I liked you better plump!" I was startled for a moment and then I realized what was happening. I was much more polite when I was fat. I allowed people to waste my time. I suffered fools, if not gladly, at least pleasantly. What my grocery man really misses is a more obsequious me. I guess I am now more sensitive about allowing people to push me around. Maybe I often let them do that when I was fat and hated myself. I have to practice the difference between being obsequious and being polite.

Friends and Relations

Before, during and after dieting, we have to be constantly on guard against sabotage from the people who are close to us, who love us, but are often unaware of the ways in which they make dieting more difficult for us. We are not the only ones who are terrified of our becoming thin; as much as those closest to us may *say* they are glad, the truth is they may be having plenty of anxieties of their own.

While I was in Durham, this was especially clear in relation to the young people. As they lost weight, some of their parents were frightened by a new kind of relationship—one in which the child would be more assertive, less dependent:

> Dan's father was on a business trip and stopped off to see him. He is the person who shamed and ridiculed Dan the most and urged him to come here. Dan said, "All he could talk about was that I needed a haircut. The next topic of conversation was how much all this was costing him. He wasn't the least impressed that I'd lost twenty pounds. He just said, 'That's a drop in the bucket—you have a long way to go.' Then he insisted that we go out to eat and *urged* me to order a steak dinner!"

All the terrors we have felt seem to be coming true when the people we love make it clear that *they* have ambivalent feelings about what we are doing—that *they* feel threatened by our struggle to become more fully alive, to realize ourselves. Even under the best of circumstances, when there has been a great deal of openness and communication, panic may set in. I knew that my husband wanted me to fulfill myself in the way I needed to, that this was the code by which he lived. In spite of that certainty, there were periods of great anxiety. I wrote:

> Wendy called today. She said, "What's the matter with Daddy? He sounds terrible. He's got the flu but he won't admit it. He also won't admit how much he misses you. He's a mess!"
>
> My mother-in-law called today. She is very worried about Larry. He's had a bad cold for three weeks. She tells me he was very susceptible to pneumonia as a child. "You know, Eda," she says, "it's all very well for you to lose weight,

but if it kills your husband, it isn't going to make you happy." At first I was so furious—I wanted to kill them all, I wanted to run away and never go back home. And then I realized that this is part of the reality I must deal with; that Larry and I must talk this out. When I'm not around, he loses any sense of time—"forgets" to eat or sleep. I cannot allow this to stop me. If I go running home now, both of us would suffer. We both want me to succeed—it would be a shared failure. I know that he wants me to stay here and also that both of us are ambivalent about it. I called my mother-in-law back and said I shared her great concern for Larry's health, and told her that if Larry was really sick, of course I would go home. I realized that she was just worried. Larry and I had a long talk on the phone. I told him how I was feeling. I told him that if he could just admit to himself that he misses me, maybe he'd get over his cold. I even sang a bit of "A Person Could Develop a Cold" from *Guys and Dolls*—the first musical comedy to suggest a psychogenic cause for colds! He finally laughed, admitted he misses me, and said he'd try to take better care of himself.

The unchanged behavior of a marriage partner seems to confirm every anxiety we ever had before we started:

Linda was terribly troubled and unhappy after going home for a week's furlough. She's reluctant to talk about it, but finally she told me that her husband was impotent. It wasn't anything new; it has been a recurring problem all through her fifteen-year marriage. They talk about getting help— therapy for him, marriage counseling for both of them— and maybe even a Johnson and Masters kind of consultation. But her husband feels such shame that he can't bring himself to do anything about it. In other ways, they seem to have a good marriage. They have no children, but they travel a lot and are partners in a successful business. She says, "I began to get fat from frustration, I guess, and then I got even fatter because I always blamed myself—if I were more attractive or sexy, it wouldn't happen. I know in my head that isn't the whole problem, but I always thought I was an ugly, unattractive, unlovable child, and when Mat fell in love with me I couldn't believe it. The impotence somehow seemed, well, as if I deserved it." Yet this had been a triumphant homecoming; she looked sensational and Mat seemed truly overjoyed for her. And the problem was worse than ever. Linda told me: "I wasn't sure I should come back here at all. What's the use? Being thin didn't make any difference, so I'll probably end up being fat again anyway."

Where there are serious problems like this one in close relationships, it is just as important to try to help our partners as ourselves. In fact, when obesity plays a part in the way in which a couple or a parent and a child relate to each other, there is absolutely no way we can hope to lose weight and not regain it unless there is a willingness on the part of other family members to find out just what is going on, and learn to communicate about their feelings. Very often sexual inadequacy is unconsciously blamed on the obese partner; when the spouse loses weight, the husband or wife has to look into his or her own needs and conflicts. It is a time of reckoning, of reassessment. Having struggled so desperately for our own right to live, we may now have to help other members of our family deal with their feelings.

Now we can try to extend the compassion we have come to feel for ourselves to the people whom we love. Instead of getting angry or frightened, we need to find ways to reassure and to encourage exploration and communication:

Joyce just came back from Atlanta for a checkup—she was here about two years ago and lost 110 pounds. It's hard to imagine, she's such a tiny lady now. She told me that when she went home, after losing all that weight, she was met at the airport by her thirty-year-old daughter, who burst into sobs and screamed, "Where is my *mother?*" "It was one helluva rotten victory!" she said.

She added: "I learned something very important at that moment. I realized that my relationship with my daughter had become much too close. I hadn't really let her grow up and away from me when I was fat. I needed all the love I could get. I realized I had exploited her, and after the first shock, she and I had some of the most honest and painful talks we had ever had. I told her I thought she needed some therapy because she was too attached to me. At first she felt even more rejected and angry. But a few months later she admitted to me that she and her husband had gone for marriage counseling. He had received several offers of better jobs over a period of years and my daughter always refused to move because she wanted to be near me. Now they have moved to Seattle. I think my losing weight was the best thing that ever happened to her."

I am convinced that a good part of the recidivism that occurs results from the fact that in subtle and unconscious ways the obese member of the family is cooperating with the sabotage, in fear of losing the relationship. Long after leaving Durham, on a speaking assignment in California, I wrote in my diary:

I looked up Fran, who had been my neighbor in the motel in Durham. She lives in a beautiful home right on the beach, about fifty miles from Los Angeles. She is much heavier now than when she first came to Durham. As soon as she got home, her husband had insisted that she cook rich, heavy meals for him. He treats her like a servant—is constantly giving her orders. If Fran were twenty or thirty years younger, I think she might have come home and gotten a divorce. But she's in her early fifties, she's never been trained for anything, she didn't go to college, she's never lived on her own and her husband is rich; she feels safe. She's being the good, obedient little girl she was trained to be as a child.

One of the lessons I learned in living with many obese people was that our feelings of self-hatred had somethimes poisoned our marriages. I wrote in my journal:

The more we talk and share our feelings, the more I realize that most of us who are fat have the unconscious feeling that there is something wrong with a spouse who could really love us! We poison the relationship with a kind of contempt. "My wife is a doll," John says, "but I keep think-ing, what is the matter with her if she can love all 280 pounds of me?"

I realize that quite unconsciously I have done the same thing. I know rationally that I am married to a brilliant, attractive, remarkable man, sought after by many other women. I know rationally that I am special too, but some-where, deep down, there has always been this seed of doubt. Feeling ugly, hating myself, I know now that I often won-dered, what is the matter with him, if he can love me? The horror of it is that this equation damages my esteem for him. If I continue to feel that he loved me *in spite of* my being overweight, I demean him as well as myself.

I am beginning to see more clearly; loving is just loving and ought to be celebrated without doubts. I think the fact that I am now proportionately thinner than he is for the first time in our married lives has forced me to examine where my self-hatred was leading us. I realize for the first time that I would love *him* no matter what he looked like; it's just so much gravy that he's wonderful-looking! But I would love him if he were fat and ugly, and that doesn't diminish *my* judgment at all! It shows I know a good thing when I see it. If that is true, then there was nothing the matter with him for loving me!

I realize I have imposed this sense of "something wrong" on any man who could love me. Like so many people, I was caught in the trap of the *Vogue* magazine perception of what is attractive. There are so many things that make people attractive inside and outside: Being cuddly, having warm and loving eyes, full and sensual lips, saying funny things, being unpredictable and always exciting, being able to roar in anger and purr in contentment and shout in exultation, being an "original," someone unique and special in a thousand ways. I *respect* people who love me now! And I am shocked to face the ways in which I denigrated *them* through my self-hatred.

As we become aware of such distortions, we begin to realize that such problems cannot be cured by merely losing weight. If we want to remain slimmer, sooner or later we have to deal with the painful question of whether or not we can change ourselves, and also whether or not there is the possibility for helping a partner to change. This is of course where some of the terror of losing weight began and we are now faced with deciding for or against our own needs. If we do not capitulate— if we make it clear that we will no longer allow the sabotage to occur—there is a good chance that others will begin to behave differently or become willing to join us in seeking professional counseling, when this seems necessary.

Sabotage in Everyday Life

We have to become increasingly sensitized as well toward ordinary thoughtlessness on the part of people on the periphery of our lives. I have been amazed at what I have observed happening in my own life. Some of it is annoying, some of it makes me angry, some of it is just funny. Here are a few examples of such occurrences that I recorded:

> We have had a series of visitors recently and it suddenly occurred to me that in the past several months we have received salt and pepper sets as gifts from three different people. That's more than I have gotten in thirty-four years of marriage! And all since I announced to the world that I'd be on a salt-free diet for the rest of my life! *Weird!*

Maxine wrote me about adjusting to being back home. She listed the comments she's been hearing. "A self-righteous aunt said, 'You better keep it off!' A friend who can't stop smoking said, 'You're much too thin now.' From a fat friend whose husband had just complimented me: 'It's just as dangerous to be too thin as to be too fat.' A friend at the golf course said, 'It's great while it lasts, but I never met anyone who didn't gain it all back.' It's wonderful to be home!"

I got an emergency call—would I come and give a speech in Chicago? Pat got stuck at the last minute and is desperate. When I said no, I was still dieting and traveling was just too difficult, she said in a slightly patronizing tone, "Well, I wouldn't want to do anything to interfere with your *health*, but you're not sick—are you just doing this for *beauty?*"

I called New York on business this morning and Bill's secretary was feeling very chatty. "We all love you just the way you are," she told me. "You shouldn't deprive yourself of the pleasures of food—life is too short. It's not necessary to be thin at your age." She's thirty and wears a size 5!

I met Dan quite by accident in an airport the other day. He yelled at me, "There's less of you to love!" I wanted to kill him on the spot. I said, "Don't you ever *dare* say that to me again—you of all people, who chase every broad who looks like Twiggy!" He left hurriedly. I don't think we will be likely to have any further conversations!

Last night Diane called to find out how I was doing. I told her I had lost thirty pounds. Her first comment was, "How will I *know* you?" That's a terrifying question, which plays right into my own anxieties. But that was minor; then she said, "Poor Larry, all the men will be chasing after you!" The implication was clear that while I was fat, there was no such danger.

Roger wrote me: "Why did you have to go to North Carolina to starve to death? You could have done it at home

and all your friends could have witnessed your disappear-
ance." Thin people seem to have some of the same fantasies
fat people have!

Letter from Kate: "I don't like the idea of your being
skinny. You might look gaunt and less inviting and warm."

Alice called. She said, "I'll be so *jealous!* Now you'll be
famous and successful *and thin!* It's almost too much to bear!"

Nadine came back from a visit home. She reported to
us how it felt to be among "civilians" again. Not good!
"Everybody congratulated me and complimented me, but
nobody believed I was really serious about staying thin.
People were constantly inviting me out to lunch and dinner,
to cocktail parties. They kept trying to entice me to have
'just one tiny drink,' or 'You must just *taste* this.' The world
is full of saboteurs," she told us.

It often felt that way, that the "enemy" was "out there," and
no one can deny that the pressures are often hard to deal with,
but ultimately we make our own choices and must hold ourselves
accountable.

One of the reasons most of us got fat in the first place is
that we allowed ourselves to be exploited. The day I left New
York for my extended stay in North Carolina, a friend blurted
out on the phone, "But you *can't* go away now—I need you!"
When and how did I become responsible? Another friend said
she would miss me too much and would come to visit me. I
said I wasn't going to allow anyone to come and she replied,
"You're right—about everyone else but me!" How did I encourage this idea of her being an exception? Before losing weight,
I allowed others to exploit me. It made me furious and depressed,
but I was never able to do anything about it. What I have had
to face is that in every case where demands were made on me,
I made the choice of what to do about it; being loved was so damned
important that I could never say no. Being loved *is* important,

but each one of us has to make choices about how much love we can give to others and still have enough left over for ourselves. I will never succeed at this task completely, but what I have learned is to recognize the signs of distress very quickly and to do something about it. If I am in the middle of working and someone calls and says, "I hate to bother you, but . . ." I tell them they may *not* bother me right now. When someone says, "You just have to learn to say no to everyone but me," I have become brave enough to say, "You're included."

Another part of being fat is that eating is a way of comforting ourselves about disappointments in other people. We satiate ourselves with food because someone has "let us down"—we expected something more and feel angry and unhappy. It is just as important not to "lay our trip" on other people as it is not to let others exploit us. After I lost weight and came back home, I wrote in my journal:

> I see so many changes in myself. I find that I am accepting a sort of *quiet*, permanent sadness where Sue is concerned. I'm no longer angry at unfulfilled expectations; rather, I am allowing the natural sadness to become a part of the fabric of my life—I am not fighting it anymore. That seems to make an enormous difference.

Nothing is more important to me than love and friendship. If I seem to be viewing it with a jaundiced eye thus far in this chapter, it is only to redress a balance. We eat too much when we feel people are eating us emotionally. If we want to stop eating too much, we have to put a limit on other people's claims.

The more we respect our own lives and selves, the more likely we are to influence others to feel the same way about themselves. Self-love is contagious! When I first decided to go to Durham, I could not anticipate that I would influence the lives of friends or relatives. One friend told me, "You have no idea how moved I am by what you are doing. It forces me to think about how

I value my life, what I need to do to fulfill myself. You are an inspiration." While I was away, several friends started dieting. One friend quit a good job for one that paid less but was more fulfilling. A relative wrote me: "Your self-imposed exile has affected me very deeply. I'm trying to care more about myself and my life."

The problem for most of us, fat or thin, is that we grew up with the mistaken notion that to be for oneself was selfish—even immoral. What many of us have had to learn is that quite the reverse is true. Once we are truly for ourselves, it becomes possible to care far more profoundly about other people. The more alert and sensitive I become to my own needs—and the more I am able to fight for what I need—the more loving and generous I want to be toward others. Resentment is banished and in its place comes a deeper compassion for others.

The Support System Is Also There

I have stressed the ways in which others make demands on us because this is a reality fat people tend to deny. But it is equally important to recognize, encourage—enjoy—the ways in which so many people help us with their love and support. We often feel used and abused because *we* find it very difficult to allow others the pleasure of being kind and thoughtful to us.

I have always had a problem taking from others; that's a characteristic common to many of us who run for the bread box! We give and give until we are angry and exhausted—but we have seldom allowed ourselves to play the role of the receiver; it embarrasses us and makes us uncomfortable. The day I left Durham, the following episode occurred:

> Barbara insisted that she wanted to drive me to the airport. She brought me a marvelous present and also insisted on taking me out to lunch. I was overwhelmed and embarrassed and started to fight with her over the check. Finally she

yelled at me, "Eda, can't you ever let anybody do anything for *you?* Do you have to be the giver all the time? Can't you allow me the pleasure of letting you know how much you have helped me, how much you mean to me?" I was shocked. She's right: I'm not a gracious taker. I allowed myself to bask in this friendship and to be grateful for her love.

I should have known better by that day of leave-taking, because for all the time I was in Durham I had been the recipient of an outpouring of love and encouragement. Looking back at those three and a half months, I realize I was being forced to learn a new skill—allowing others to take care of me and letting them know I was grateful. I wrote in my journal:

My room looks like a hothouse or a nursery! I feel overwhelmed by such an outpouring of loving messages. Today an enormous floral arrangement arrived: "Some Spring Love to Keep You Warm from Bill and Susie." When I came in and found it, I was shivering and freezing from walking home from the Rice House. I felt flooded by warmth—it was the perfect message. Two days ago, a veritable *tree* arrived from my favorite editor: "For a little help with your loneliness. Love, David." I feel overwhelmed by such loving attention. It embarrasses me. I must learn to accept it and enjoy it.

Got a cute birthday card from my father today. There was some rice in the envelope and the message: "Confucius say you have now entered the Rice Age."

The mail helps so much. Especially funny letters. One today from darling Bil Baird, a charming and mischievous elf, who wrote me: "This thing can be carried too far. A journalist friend of mine reduced so much that his fingers used to get stuck between the typewriter keys."

People seem to want to reassure me that they loved me fat! Phyllis wrote today: "I always understood your pain—

but since I loved you so much, you always looked good to me."

I came into lunch wearing new slacks and Dick looked at me appreciatively and said, "Goodbye, fat lady!" He was genuinely pleased and happy for me. It was really a way of confirming my own inner declaration—a sensitive and caring response. He knows what hard work it is. I realize now that before, I never expected to be noticed. Maybe now I will begin to expect to be treated with more courtesy, attention and appreciation.

How complicated the human condition! We need love and recognition, and yet somehow we fear it. We want to help other people and yet we often do so at the price of denying help to ourselves. It is so hard to find a balance and yet that is the task we must set for ourselves. If we won't care for ourselves, nobody else can do it for us. And yet others *do* make a difference. I think one of the most loving gestures of farewell, when I left New York to go to Durham, came from a friend who said, "Give me a *last fat hug!*" It was a message of love for me the way I was, with an acceptance of *my* need to change.

8

Fat No More: Dealing with Change

A major aspect of the terror of becoming thinner is that when we change, the attitudes of others whom we care about will change toward us. By the time you are no longer fat, your anxieties and fantasies may well have returned in full force and must be reckoned with. The struggle continues; another round of self-searching and self-testing that sometimes makes the preliminary battle of the bulges seem like child's play. It is, of course, the reason why most people gain all the weight back. But the war can be won.

When I arrived in Durham, I was convinced that all my really tough problems were over: I understood the multitude of complex reasons why I had never been able to sustain a weight loss and the rest would just be a mechanical problem. I felt very superior to my fellow dieters: poor things, so few of them understood the neurotic reasons for their obesity, but I did, and that would make all the difference. My smug sense of superiority lasted about a day and a half. What I had to learn the hard way was that I would have to deal with my terrors in an entirely new way because now I was *really changing*. We may have had a *distorted* self-image while we were fat, but a *changing* self-image can blow your mind completely!

Who the Hell Am I?

No one sees him- or herself with genuine objectivity. What each of us sees in the mirror is based on the inner distortions and confusions that began to develop when we were young children. We saw ourselves as we thought our parents saw us, and later as we thought our peers saw us. Neither criterion was particularly useful or accurate. But most of all, we see ourselves through our own confused feelings. I suspect that the reason people enjoy looking at themselves in distorted mirrors at amusement parks is that they are seeing themselves as they think they really are! The distorted image somehow seems more real than what one sees in an ordinary mirror.

However we see our selves, this self-image is of vital importance—it colors everything we do and feel. When there is a rapid and dramatic weight loss, the psychological impact can be cataclysmic. I wrote in my Durham journal:

> My first lesson in Durham was that losing too much weight too quickly can cause severe psychological stress. One's body image affects every aspect of one's life. My immediate impression of the dieters staying at the motel is that they are enormously kind to each other. That's why Terry stands out like a sore thumb. Everybody seems to dislike her intensely. She seems to be narcissistic and hypochondriacal—constantly asking for special attention from everyone at the motel as well as from the medical staff at the hospital.
>
> One of the other women told me, "Don't pay any attention to Terry." What fascinates me is that Terry is so universally hated. I've been witnessing so many acts of compassion and

tenderness between people that it seems out of character for this place.

[Two weeks later] Terry took me to her room and she began telling me about herself. She has lost 180 pounds in eighteen months! The doctors had told her that she could go home but she felt too weak and sick. She knew there was something seriously wrong with her, but the doctors wouldn't tell her what it was. Then she showed me her "before" picture. Here was this thin, gaunt woman in front of me and the picture seemed to be someone else altogether—a mountain of flesh. *There was literally no way in which to identify that this was the same woman.*

I realized that she was suffering from an almost psychotic hypochondriasis and that her terrible fears of sickness and dying were caused by her total loss of any sense of who she was. In some ways I think she felt she had already died; becoming preoccupied with illness was a way of warding off that absence of self.

A few weeks later one of the doctors told me about a woman whom they wanted to discharge, but who would not go home. She lived in New York and the doctor wondered if I could refer her to a psychiatrist there. I wrote:

Betty had lost eighty-five pounds in six months. She is terrified that she is dying of cancer. "Something is eating away at me," she told me. "I know it—it's eating and growing, eating and growing."

It is mind-blowing to realize how much *the way we look* determines whether or not we know *who we are*. It's very frightening. But I think part of the problem for Terry and Betty was that nothing had changed *except* their size; neither had dealt at all with the problems that had got them there in the first place. Old feelings of self-hatred and the need for self-punishment can begin to take new forms as we lose our old self-images. Having lost weight without any changes in attitudes and feelings, Terry and Betty had needed to find some new form of self-torture—such as the fear of dying. Neither one was enjoying being thin. They didn't seem to want to buy beautiful clothes, and they had no desire to go on with their lives. Their bodies belonged to strangers, and in their terror they were hanging on with desperation to what was familiar to them—self-hatred and self-punishment.

How do any of us know who we are? Many of the dimensions of our self-image are internalized, unconscious attitudes from earliest childhood. To some degree we recognize ourselves in terms of ideas, thoughts, attitudes, behavior and relationships. But at the deepest and most primitive level, we are really our bodies—our physical selves. A sudden and radical change in the very structure of our being can and does cause tremendous disruption and a sense of terrifying turmoil.

The total personality disruption that I saw in Terry and Betty was, of course, extreme—but it was the beginning of my learning how difficult it would be to deal with changes in my own appearance. I was better prepared than they, and the physical changes would be less dramatic since I had less weight to lose, but their stories helped to prepare me for the identity crisis I found myself living through. I began to realize just how important my long period of introspection, my quest for self-understanding, had been; at least "I knew the ropes" for dealing with my feelings—and a lot of the traps.

For example, at one point I said to Terry, "God, it must be such a terrible shock to look so different!" She smiled sweetly and said, "Oh, no, not at all; it's wonderful. The only problem now is that I'm not well." She had had every possible medical test and all were negative, but she clung to this explanation of her difficulties. Consciously she talked about how proud she felt, how much she looked forward to "getting well" and returning to her job, but when she talked about her former life it was as if she was talking about another person, not in the room with us. She was split off from herself and didn't even know it. Observing her dilemma helped prepare me for my own aberrations.

As the Image Changes

After losing thirty-five pounds, I wrote in my journal:

> With fear and trembling I put on my new bathing suit and went to the motel pool this afternoon. Half of me wanted somebody to notice and the other half was hoping no one would pay any attention. Marty, Josh and Helen were there and they all noticed and made a fuss over me. I was delighted and relieved. It is so good to have a safe place to try myself on for my new size!
>
> I'm practicing for what will happen when the difference is noticed by everyone who knew me before. I'm trying to learn to be gracious and happy and to talk about it easily, instead of hiding.

In order to deal with a changing self-image, I became preoccupied with my appearance:

> I find myself examining myself in the mirror more and more, sensitive to every physical flaw. I noticed today that my chin is sort of sagging. I have more wrinkles all over—it's disgusting. My face looks smaller. I feel as if I am looking at a child's face in the mirror. Because I used to feel fat and unattractive, I ignored external surfaces—in myself and in everybody else. Am I going to become a superficial person, only interested in how people look? How *I* look? I'll lose all respect for myself if this mirror-gazing doesn't stop!

One of the reasons most people gain all the weight back is that they get very frightened when they begin to behave in slightly crazy ways—and they retreat and regress. But if you know *why* you're getting a little peculiar, you can tolerate this phase and get through it.

Each of us seems to develop a unique and individual style of nuttiness:

> This morning I took Doris shopping. All her clothes are too big, and she's used to wearing heavy corsets. We bought some bras and panties, and she was so excited to see herself in them that she strutted about the dressing room, shouting—she even started to go into the lingerie department to show the salesladies! I had to corral her like a five-year-old! She's forty-nine years old, and I had to act like her mother, telling her that the store has rules against people running about in bras and panties! The way she seems to be handling a lot of her anxiety is by regressing to being a little girl—a place to try to find a sense of identity all over again.

Annie told me this story:

> "After I'd lost all that weight, I went home and went to the most exclusive dress shop in town to buy myself an original—a designer dress. Never in my life had it ever occurred to me that I would become a size 6 and be able to buy such a dress. I tried on one dress after the other. I became terribly depressed. I hated myself in every one of them. The saleslady was going crazy—these were the most gorgeous, expensive clothes to be found anywhere, and all I kept saying was, No, this makes me look too fat! After this had been going on for about half an hour, the saleslady said, 'I hope this question won't offend you, but have you lost a great deal of weight recently?' I was very startled and asked her how she knew. She told me that she had waited on several other customers in recent months who were trying on sixes and eights, and none of them bought a dress because they saw themselves as fat, no matter what they put on. She had discovered that in every case they had come from a nearby spa, where they had all lost a great deal of weight."

The most frightening experience I had in the process of discovering and accepting a new self-image occurred one afternoon at a theater. I'd gone into the ladies' room, where there was a mirror the length of the wall. About ten women were standing in front of it, combing their hair, fixing their makeup. I looked into the mirror, and for a split second I could not identify which one of the women in that mirror was *me*. I laughed about it when I reported it to my husband—it seemed very funny. For about five minutes. Then the creeping terror was back. How could I stay thin if I didn't know who I was? I am sure this loss of a sense of identity accounts for a major portion of the recidivism among dieters.

Being aware of what was happening made all the difference. If this episode had occurred ten years ago, I would have been so scared I would have rushed from the theater to the nearest ice cream parlor.

As I realized how difficult the readjustment was, it occurred to me that what we formerly fat people need is some sort of decompression chamber, so we don't get the bends when we see our "before" and "after" pictures—a "halfway house" where we could live without mirrors for a couple of months. But in the absence of such a resource, we just have to watch what is happening to us and understand that it is normal and natural to be shook up by a brand-new body.

It is not merely that we *look* different; other things change too, adding to feelings of shock, discomfort, insecurity. Here are a few samples of these kinds of experiences as I recorded them in my journal:

> It is seventeen degrees out today and the wind is blowing in gusts up to thirty miles per hour. Although I put on about three layers of clothing, I still felt as if there was nothing between my poor bones and the Arctic Circle! I'm freezing most of the time. *No insulation!* I still have more fat padding than my really thin friends—but it's the change that makes it feel this way.

When I get cold, I put on a sweater; I also bought a small electric heater for my office. I'm buying woolen dresses. I'm accommodating myself to biological changes and trying not to feel frightened by them!

Maria was very comforting to me today. I said I felt as if all the seats in all the movie theaters in New York had suddenly sprung; I just can't sit without feeling uncomfortable and squirming a lot. I also find that if I half lie–half sit in bed to read for any length of time, my coccyx begins to hurt like hell. Maria assured me this is not old age, it is just the price one pays for being thinner.

Something must have happened, if I'm going home in a *belted* coat! Never had one before in my whole life!

I went to a little dress shop in my neighborhood today, figuring I'd treat myself to one more size 14 before waiting to lose more weight. But I bought a size 12! I'm in a state of shock; I don't *know* an Eda who could wear a size 12. It has to be a mistake. I tried on twenty dresses, just to be sure they weren't mislabeled! I also bought a pair of high-heeled shoes! First time in about thirty years. I felt terribly clumsy—it was like the first time I ever bought a pair when I was a teen-ager, and I wobble around on them.

Another surprise—something I hadn't thought about or anticipated: it is so much roomier in a double bed! I curl up into such a small, snug ball!

The most simple routines, things that one has always done quite unconsciously, change—often long before we are aware of it. The way one bends down to tie a shoelace is different; squeezing past the refrigerator isn't squeezing anymore. The realization that one has changed without even being conscious of the change is startling, and each formerly obese person has his or her own special adjustments to make.

I think I was able to see more clearly what was happening to me and other formerly fat people when a friend who is a therapist told me that one of his patients had lost fifty pounds and seemed to feel peculiar and uneasy. Fred told her that she was "rattling around in her space." He feels that we develop an unconscious sense of how much space we fill and that his patient wasn't "filling her space" any longer. Fred told me that this concept seemed to help his patient—and it certainly rang a bell with me.

It would be fine if we could lose weight so gradually that we could become accustomed to ourselves more easily. But some of us can't do it that way, at least in the beginning. What I discovered was that a time arrived when I was accustomed to my new body—and even ready to go on to lose more weight:

> For the past couple of weeks, I've found myself feeling fat again. I look in the mirror, wearing a size 12, and see a size 18 woman. I am beginning to feel uncomfortable, my movements somehow heavy again. The remaining bulges are really bothering me. Yesterday I went back on rice, fruit and vegetables. I seem ready to lose another ten or fifteen pounds. My image of myself has had time to change. Now that the major weight loss has been accomplished, I can consciously watch myself and never go faster than I am ready to go. I no longer feel strange; I don't feel thin: I don't feel different from what I was before. It is as if I have settled into this body, know it, *am* it—and that makes it possible to go on again. Without anxiety, without loss of identity.

The Stranger in the Body

A further inevitable complication is that your personality is undergoing major changes as well as your body. It's a tossup which is more frightening—the new image in the mirror or the changed person looking at that image. I had to continue to notice what was happening to me, so that I could deal with my feelings. Lack of awareness about what is happening is what leads back to the refrigerator.

It was a great shock for me to discover that other people were treating me differently. At first I assumed they were reacting to my changed appearance, but after awhile I had to begin to face the fact that *I* was behaving differently too.

Had lunch with Sam today—all dressed up in my size 12 Halston pants suit. He's twenty years younger than I am, and our relationship has almost been mother and son—at least, I was sort of an "authority figure" in our work relationship. When I took off my coat he exclaimed, "Hey, you've really got terrific boobs!" I thought I'd pass out and sink right through the floor. In an instant he had changed our roles with each other. It embarrassed the hell out of me—but I liked it!

Part of what makes it so damned hard is what other people do and say. The other day, Allen called; he hasn't seen me since I lost all the weight. He's a man I don't know terribly well, but we are colleagues and like each other. "I've *got* to see you!" he said. "I bet you're so sexy that I won't be able to keep my hands off you!" My immediate reaction was terror and then anger. The terror is: What will I do if that's true? And my anger is: I was "sexy" when I was fat—how come he didn't know that? Finally he laughed and added, "You will never be the girl for assignations!" What does *he* know? What do *I* know? I want to be old—really old and decrepit—so this whole subject never comes up in conversation.

Then there was the plumber who came to turn off the water in our summer home. We have seen each other a few times each summer for the past four years. He told Larry: "You better watch out! You might lose her, now that she's so sexy! I know a couple where the man was very fat. He lost almost a hundred pounds, and the next thing we knew, he ran away with a young chick and left his wife!"

I assured him that there was no chance of that. Larry just laughed and said he wasn't worried. Again the terror and the anger: am I in danger of becoming wanton? And why is it that everybody thinks fat is unsexy and thin is sexy? But I know that it isn't just that I look different. My attitude is different too. I wonder who I was before? I am constantly being reminded that I *did* hide behind the fat. And often want to again.

The fantasy that I would become a wanton woman if I got thin was only half wrong; I didn't develop nymphomaniacal qualities, but sex certainly became more of an issue. I wrote in my journal:

It is perfectly clear that I am crazy; I don't know what I want, that's for sure. When strange men are attentive or flirtatious, I can be very nasty one minute, and the next I'm enjoying it thoroughly. What happens is that if a man invites me for a drink, or offers to help me carry a package, or holds a door open for me, my first reaction is: "Why didn't you treat me this way when I was fat, you bastard!" I am the same person, I tell myself. But sooner or later the truth dawns on me. It is true that strange men are more likely to start a conversation now, but it is not entirely due to my weight loss; *my attitude is different.* It is true that most men, having been programmed to believe fat is ugly, make fewer overtures to fat women, but if I were merely thinner, no man would start a conversation with me if I were as aloof to strange men as I used to be. I allow myself the pleasure of the company of strange men now.

So much of the content of feelings about sex and over-weight is unconscious—for thin people too. Out of the clear blue sky, Bruce asks on the telephone, "Hey, listen, if you keep losing weight, what am I going to do about you?" At first I didn't have any idea what he meant, and when I asked, he got embarrassed and changed the subject abruptly. I think it was something that just came out of his unconscious; if I'm thin, and we are such close friends, and love each other already—will it mean that even though we are both happily married, there will be some different content in our relationship? What he is saying is that as long as I was fat, the relationship felt safe. I guess that's true for both of us!

I had not anticipated the kinds of feelings—the dramatic adjustments—that were in store for me after I had lost weight, but when they occurred, I was already accustomed to analyzing my feelings and giving myself the comforting, the compassion, I needed. By going through the process of self-examination over and over again, I was able to ride out the most dramatic period of change. I wrote in my Durham journal:

> Last night there was a magnificent performance of *La Bohème* on PBS. At supper Mark reminded me that it was going to be on. He's another opera buff, and we had fun talking about some of our "peak experiences" at memorable performances of operas. During the first intermission he phoned me from his room to see how I was enjoying it.
>
> Pavarotti was Rodolfo, and I was ecstatic. So was Mark. Without thinking, I said, "Hey, why don't you come and listen in my room? We can both cry and clap and have a fine time!" Mark is very shy—a relatively new widower, still uneasy about women, and he said no, but I had the feeling he was sorry he couldn't say yes. After we hung up, I was amazed at what I had done. I never would have taken a risk like that, thirty pounds ago; I would have been too afraid of rejection. He's a nice man; it was his loss, not mine. It would have been fun to listen together—and an innocent pleasure for both of us. I don't feel rejected and the music was magnificent—and I am *changing!*

It is especially difficult to deal with expectations or fantasies we never even knew we had. I wrote in my journal:

> Today a nurse who is a patient here told me, "I thought everyone would notice me and fall in love with me, I'd

be so gorgeous. You know what happened? When I was fat I got a lot more attention; I was the only fat nurse, so I was known as "that fat nurse." Now I'm just like every-body else and nobody notices me or knows who I am!"

Today Joan and Sylvia were agreeing that they had each had a secret illusion that underneath all the layers of flab was the most beautiful woman in all the world. The reality of being attractive middle-aged ladies causes them periods of great depression—and cheating.

Changes in sexual feelings and behavior are often the most difficult to deal with—just as they were often what we worried about the most long before we lost weight. Some people discover that the fat was a shield against libidinal drives they were keeping "under cover"; as the weight came off, they began to enjoy a liberated sensuality. Others became frightened. Still others were surprised by totally unexpected responses. After I'd returned home, a fellow dieter, Laura, wrote me:

> Remember the time when we both realized how much colder we were? Well, much to my surprise, I seem to be frigid on the inside as well as on the outside. When I went home Sally and Rosemary gave me a going-home present—a sexy size 16 nightgown. It had the desired effect on Randy, but you know what? *I didn't feel a thing.* The same thing the next night. When I wore a size 24½ I was dynamite! It's scaring the shit out of me. Like I'm a piece of stone. By yesterday I was so upset that I spent the whole day cleaning the house. I got a backache and was exhausted by the time we went to bed. It wasn't even just no feeling—I didn't even *like* it anymore. So what do I do now, Mrs. Shrink???

For all the men and women who went on to enjoy a freer and more fulfilling sex life after losing weight, there were an equal number who seemed to be having less fun than ever before. I wrote to Laura:

First of all, cheer up; you've got lots of company! It seems to be a very common reaction. I don't know if this will be any help, but here is what occurs to me: Being thin makes a lot of us feel that we are "bad girls." Sexual pleasure would confirm that judgment and make us feel guilty. Being fat was so much punishment that we didn't have to also deprive ourselves of sex. We feel unconsciously that we can't possibly have both—being thin *and* sensual; we can't allow ourselves to have *nothing to suffer about!* Remember what we did when we were freezing in Durham? We bought scarves and woolen hats and heavy sweaters, and allowed ourselves time to adjust. Maybe it's the same sort of thing with sexual frigidity. If it's something new and unexpected, maybe you just have to relax and accept it for a while as another part of the period of adjustment.

I found that the one thing that was most helpful to me was to constantly remind myself that I was *in process;* that I must not be impatient with myself; that I must *allow* change rather than *force* it. And if I got a little peculiar from time to time, that was only natural under the circumstances. One has to learn to just *let things happen*—roll with the waves, not fight them.

A Period of Mourning

Nothing that happened during the whole period of dieting shocked me so completely as the discovery that I could not give up my fat self (or the neuroses involved therein) without a decent burial. I think it turned out to be my most important and dramatic insight about why we gain weight back; it is because we have not taken the time to mourn for someone of great importance—our fat self. I wrote in my journal:

> Forty pounds off as of today!!!! I went to the fanciest department store in town to celebrate and bought a blouse and slacks. The image in the store mirror was almost unrecogniz-

able—and beautiful! After shopping, I began walking to
the Rice House for lunch. I felt victorious and excited and
terribly happy. I kept thinking about that image in the mirror. This was someone new, a stranger—where am *I?*

Halfway to lunch, my exultant mood seemed to slip away
quite suddenly. I began to feel very sad, and could not figure
out why. Then something very strange happened: I found
myself weeping—in a state of mourning for "Fat Eda!" That
person was *me* for at least forty-five of my fifty-four years—
she brought me here—but she's going to die here. *She willed
her own death.*

Suddenly I was overwhelmed with love and grief. The
fat person I was suffered so much and tried so hard! She
went on and on, inexorably in search of answers, through
years of psychotherapy, through diet after diet—searching,
searching, never giving up—and then making the final sacri-
fice, to die here, so that someone new could live. "Thin
Eda"—who will she be? Will I like her? It is terrifying.
The old self is safe, familiar, although full of pain; the new
is strange—wonderful but frightening. I feel a wave of love
for that self I am leaving forever. She tried her best to take
care of me—she brought me to this place—she saved my
life.

She was not a bad person. She was not lazy or weak.
She suffered so much pain. I feel as if I can't let go so
easily. If I am suddenly too delighted with myself, I will
be avoiding something of equal importance. There is a kind
of death going on here, and I must pay attention to it.

About six weeks later, having lost fifty pounds, I was ready
to go home. It was time for another complete medical checkup
at the Duke University Medical Diagnostic Clinic. I wrote:

In between the various tests at the clinic, I went for a walk
in the Duke Gardens. It is one of the most beautiful places
I've ever seen, especially at this time of year, with all the
flowering trees in bloom. I felt quiet and sad—I guess I'm

frightened about leaving in a few days, wondering what will happen to me at home. I sat down on a tree stump to look at the woods and watch the birds—all busy building their nests, I guess.

I remember my first terrifying day here—the strangeness, not knowing what it would be like, whether or not I'd suc-ceed. Suddenly I felt terribly proud of myself. How brave I was to have come! And then a great wave of sadness, which at first I couldn't identify, until suddenly I thought of my mother—and burst into tears. How much I wish she could have known what I have done! With all the neu-rotic strains between us on the subject of dieting, she loved me more than anyone else could ever love me—no matter how many difficulties there may have been, the relationship was still the most profound and essential one. She would be glad, and she would be proud of me. How I wish I could have done it while she was alive. Nostalgia, regrets, pain—all mixed in with my sense of victory.

I also found myself mourning for the process and the place where it had occurred:

It shocks me—such a totally unexpected reaction—but I feel terrible about leaving this place! It's been so desperately important to me—such a turning point in my life. It took my full attention. I have become totally absorbed in myself and my surroundings, noticing every flower, every tree, all the plants and birds that one doesn't see farther north. The attachment is one of the most profound I have ever felt for a place. I'm so thankful that I came—and that I stayed. The living experience has been so intense that I feel a deep emotional attachment to "my fat people"; we are a clan. I've seen so much suffering and so much courage. A place and people I will never forget.

[The next day] Another day, more tests, another walk through the gardens. It's the hardest time of year to leave because it is so beautiful right now. I feel waves of sadness and loss. All along, I thought I'd be dying to leave—that it would be like escaping from prison—but it isn't like that at all. I have everything to go home for: a husband I love, work that I love, wonderful friends, an interesting and adventurous life. If I feel the pull to stay in this safe, known, needed haven, how much more this must be true of people who must face great problems when they leave!

I am *leaving part of myself here.* I never thought of that before—except once at the time I'd lost forty pounds and experienced the first sense of mourning for "Fat Eda." Now I am overwhelmed by a sense of loss. After hating myself for so many years, it seems incredible, but "Fat Eda," the self I have been for almost all of my life, is the person who suffered, who struggled, who finally, in desperation, brought me here—only to disappear, to *die!* She is gone forever. I am a stranger to myself.

I feel like writing myself a letter:

Most Beloved Fat Self:

Thank you for your courage and your love—enough to die and let me live. You suffered so much pain and you tried so hard; it has been such a struggle—as far back as memory—the hunger, the desperate efforts at control, the torment of self-consciousness and self-loathing. Always hoping, always trying, *working* so hard to change— and the failing, over and over again. The shame and frustration and disappointment. Thank you, dear friend, for caring so much and finally letting me go. I'll never, ever forget you. I will always care passionately for the suffering of others who are fat. I want to help them. I want to send out a message of caring—hope. We are together forever, in memory.

And finally, the day of departure:

In three and a half months I have accumulated so much stuff that getting home was a gigantic problem. My new clothes, the typewriter, my notes—it was a tremendous load. Larry didn't offer to meet me at the airport and I was furious. When I said, "I'm going to have so much junk," he said I should get a porter to help me. I was so angry that on the trip home I began to eat an absolutely ghastly sandwich that was served on the plane; I hadn't done that on a single flight back or forth before. When I got to the airport, it was mobbed and I had to wait a long time for my baggage. I couldn't find anyone to help me, and had to make three trips, running back and forth, to the taxi stand. By this time I felt so sorry for myself and so furious at Larry that I was practically in tears. When I finally hauled myself and all my belongings into the apartment, I was in a rage, and began screaming and crying. Larry looked very puzzled. "All you had to do was ask me!" he said—and of course he was perfectly right. Why didn't I ask him? Some strange need for him to understand without being asked.

I yelled a lot; after all I've been through, after coming down to visit me, after managing to get along on his own for such a long time, couldn't he spend one lousy hour helping me to get home? In addition, tomorrow he's going out of town for a meeting, and while I knew he couldn't help the timing, that made me mad too. By this time I was bawling my head off. Larry looked confused and contrite. No, he hadn't realized what an emotional experience coming home would be. He was sorry he hadn't understood. Suddenly I was screaming, *"Don't you realize I left someone I loved down there? Don't you realize I'll never see her again? That was me!"* And then the floodgates opened, and I wept and wept. Larry said very quietly: *"Of course.* Why didn't I think of that? *You are in mourning."* It is absolutely true. It is the kind of grief one feels at the death of a loved one. Crashing waves of pain, all-enveloping. "You're right! You're right!" I howled. *"Homage must be paid!* She can't just be forgotten! There must be some kind of memorial service." Very quietly Larry suggested, "You can dedicate your book to her."

Changing Relationships

Larry had been working intensely on his own psychological problems. Both of us were feeling better, working more creatively, loving each other more profoundly than ever before. One day when we were talking about all this, I suddenly heard myself saying, "Will we still love each other without our neuroses? Without feeling emotionally crippled?" We were both shocked. But it seemed to be a question we had to face.

We fall in love for a multitude of reasons. Partly because someone else sees the dream of what we want to be—the best we have in us. But we also fall in love because whatever feeling of self-hatred we may have will be assuaged: "Let me choose someone who is as damaged as I am because then we will cling to each other." We become accustomed not only to our own pain but to our partner's as well. Part of each of us says to our partner, "Hurray for you—become your most marvelous and special self!" But another inner voice says, "Be weak, be crippled; if you get too strong you might leave me; you might want someone better than me."

Larry and I are very lucky; we understand the inner terror of being whole and the reluctance to change—even when it means giving up pain and crippling. It is the "known," and we must now deal with something new and strange. Larry said, "I know it's a struggle, but I think we can learn to live without suffering!"

If we allow ourselves a period of mourning, a reintegration begins to take place. I no longer feel that sense of having to be split into two different people. Now, looking back a few years later, the idea that I had to say goodbye to my fat self seems unreal—even a little crazy. I am one person again—my past blending with my present self, a whole person looking to the future. Without that period of mourning, I don't believe this would have happened. It was true for those others whom I met in Durham who seemed to understand the necessity of this process. I had talked at length with one friend there, while we were both dealing with these feelings. We needed to feel sad and mournful before we could feel exultant and whole:

> Got a letter from Eleanor today. She wrote: "Dr. Kempner went away on vacation. While he was gone, I went off insulin completely, and got to the point where I could walk three miles a day! I went to a hair stylist and a makeup consultant at a department store. When Dr. Kempner came back, he didn't recognize me. When I told him who I was, he said, 'Gott in Himmel!' I loved every moment of it. I wear a size 5 now. You and I know why I'm making it; we shared our feelings of grief—we let it all happen—and now that it's over, we are home free!"

How wonderful change becomes when we allow ourselves to experience it fully! It can be an adventure in which fear is accepted as part of the fabric of life, so that joy and exultation can also be felt profoundly. We never get one without the other. The day after I returned home, a friend sent me a beautiful bouquet. The note with it said: "Welcome home, Columbus! You have had a good voyage—thank you for bringing the spice of life back to New York!"

What a gift that was! It made me realize that I had been an explorer moving into strange, uncharted, mysterious territory—and that I had found my way back home.

Change had been my friend—*for* me, not against me. I could now begin to enjoy other people's surprise and confusion. One day on a bus, a woman said, "Pardon me, but are you related to Eda LeShan?" A few days later, I got stuck in an elevator with a lady who said, "Has anyone ever told you that your voice is like Eda LeShan's?" And then there was the delicious (a perfect choice of words!) moment when I was standing in line at a movie theater and a man said, "My wife wants me to ask you: Are you now, or have you ever been, Eda LeShan?"

The comment I loved best came from a New Englander, a friend who fits the stereotype—laconic, never wasting a word, gets right to the point. He just looked at me, smiled and said, "Hi, Slim!"

9

What's So Great About Not Being Fat?

No one is ever happy all the time. The most malevolent fable we were ever told as children was that if we were good, we would live happily ever after. The fact that more than 90 percent of those who lose weight gain it back only goes to show that we all were brainwashed into believing such nonsense. You lose the weight—and then you wait: A handsome prince or a beautiful princess will suddenly appear by magic, and you will never be lonely again. Tomorrow you will be offered the perfect job at double your present pay. Having been so virtuous in losing weight, you *deserve* to get rich, be successful, have an easier time. Now shoelaces won't break, panty hose won't run, the supermarket checker won't cheat, the cleaners won't ruin your best slacks, the children will never get sick and will always behave perfectly, the traffic light won't change just as you get ready to cross the street, taxes will go down and your car will never need a new carburetor. *Forget it!* Whatever one's problems may have been— big or little—getting thinner isn't going to make any of them disappear. How you handle them, what you do about them, will change if your attitude toward yourself has changed—but nobody—ever—lives happily ever after. A fellow dieter recently wrote me: "When people ask me if I'm happier now, I say, No, but I've learned that everybody is as unhappy as I am!" Another friend wrote: "I'm thinner, not happier; I'm happy I'm thinner—but that's a different thing altogether." However, I know that it is not enough to say that all a diet does is take off weight. There *is* a difference, and I need to understand it before I can let go.

Losing weight didn't transform me into a beautiful young woman; it didn't make writing any easier; I've been having problems with my gall bladder and bursitis in my arm and neck that keep me awake nights. The problems and eccentricities of the people I care about did not disappear. Life has gone on presenting me with at least one major crisis per week. What was so important about losing weight? Does it really matter?

Nurturing the Child Within

In this morning's mail there were three requests for me to give speeches. They were all from friends and all for good causes. I said no to all of them. In the process of getting ready to lose weight and living through the experience of doing it, *I learned to care for my own life*. A year ago I would have said yes to all three requests; if I had turned down any of them, I would have felt awash in guilt. While traveling to wherever I might have gone, I would have stuffed myself with food to control my anger at myself as well as to give myself comfort for doing what I hated doing. If I had refused the assignments and stayed home, I would have eaten too much, to punish myself for not being a "good person."

It may seem like a small issue—giving a speech—but it is not. I'm very good at it; I've been doing it for about thirty years. For at least twenty years I have fought against the exhaustion of modern travel, hated those damned motel and hotel rooms which all look alike, the relating to hundreds of people, the plane delays, the traffic jams, the missing reservations, the small talk with strangers, the prespeech committee dinner parties where I feel obliged to be entertaining. The reason I began to hate lecturing is that about twenty years ago I began to write. It turned out to be the thing I was born to do. Continuing to give speeches seemed necessary at first for financial reasons and later in order for me to continue to think of myself as a "good person."

Losing weight and keeping it off was only a small part of a much bigger war. The real struggle was to become myself and to nourish my own soul. Deep inside there had always been a small child begging for my attention, wanting to live, to create, to be herself. All I gave her was food. Now I give her love.

In all my books and articles and on television I have tried to encourage people to nurture the child inside themselves, to find their own special music. I have assured all who would listen that by becoming themselves they would be giving more to the world, not less. I now try to practice what I preach! When I write letters refusing to give speeches; when I tell people on the telephone I can't help them; when I run away to write instead of reading the thirty books on my desk from publishers who want advance comments—I am not running away from life and responsibility. I am running toward my most essential responsibility—to be my most special self.

The truth of the matter is that my books get better the less I force myself to do other things. Writing is my natural and necessary avenue of communication, and the more I focus on that, purify it, the more of a contribution I make. Instead of scattering myself and wasting my energy, I bring a new and fresh total attention to my work. It is not that I am callous or that I don't care; rather, I realize that I have only this one tiny lifetime—diminishing so rapidly I cannot bear it—and if I nurture myself, I will be able to give the most to others. All I can really contribute is to try to be myself.

Losing weight was a peripheral bonus to the more important achievement of reaching a point of such personal self-acceptance that I don't want to be anyone but myself.

Before you even think about going on a diet and losing weight once and for all, you will have to begin to care for yourself. Stop tormenting that poor suffering person who is you. Stop hating, punishing this precious creature who is in such pain. At least try to be *almost* as kind and compassionate to your inner child as you would want to be to any other child! How shocking it is that we are so much more gentle and sensitive and responsible toward others than we are toward ourselves.

There is a starving child inside you—*starving for love* that no one else can give. The hunger can never be assuaged by a parent's love or a spouse's love or a child's love. It has to be *your* love; nothing else will do. Now is the time to look inside your soul, break through that barrier of flesh which hides what frightens you so much and allow yourself to hear that inner child crying for your solicitude and your love—and *pay attention.*

All babies are beautiful—new and vulnerable and just beginning. Inside each tiny human person is such a wealth of possibilities. How tragic it is that so much of what is there is wasted by the stupidities and agonies of the life into which each of us is born. We become crippled so soon—sometimes by neglect, sometimes by demands and expectations—by grownups who were once crippled themselves. Can you let it stop with you, in your life? If you can, you will be able to nurture others far more genuinely than ever before. You will *not* become cruel or selfish or thoughtless. You will become *yourself,* and there is an exultation in that discovery that will produce a generosity of spirit and a compassion for others far exceeding your wildest expectations.

Nothing Has Changed—and Everything Has Changed

Just before I left North Carolina, a woman who had arrived the same day as I came over to say goodbye:

> I was so touched because it seemed as if Peggy wanted to tell me something very important—some message for others. She said: "Eda, don't remember me as a person who lost fifty-five pounds. Remember me the way I was on that first day, when I was so scared and hysterical, so sure I'd never last a week. When you write your book, remember me as someone who *grew up*. Before I came here I had never done anything entirely on my own. I went straight from my parents' home into marriage. In my whole life it had never occurred to me that I could take care of myself. I learned I could deal with loneliness and being homesick; I found I could make friends, be hungry without eating, force myself to walk and do exercises even when I hated it. I have confidence in myself; I like myself. I could live alone if I had to. I can talk to other people about my feelings. I have let go of my children. I came here a sick caterpillar and now I'm a beautiful butterfly—with *wings!*"

A few weeks ago I had a perfectly terrible day; everything had gone wrong. There were all kinds of family emergencies demanding my attention; I'd written twenty-five pages in the morning and thrown them all out in the afternoon; I'd had a painful argument with a friend; my husband was preoccupied with problems of his own and seemed distant and far away. I tried to go to bed early that night, feeling exhausted, but I slept fitfully, and spent half the night pacing around the apartment, taking too many trips to the refrigerator.

By making enough noise, I finally woke up Larry, and as soon as I had his attention I began to cry. *"What's so great about being thin?"* I yelled. "I'm miserable, worried, upset, frustrated, angry, depressed. This so-called victory is ashes in my mouth—and my only comfort is that as far as I know, ashes aren't fattening!"

We talked for a long time. I agreed that I felt better and enjoyed the way I looked. Yes, I had reached a point in my psychological development where I no longer needed or wanted to be fat and was not afraid it would ever happen again. Yes, I had discovered I still had the same priorities and values and I still made my own choices. But somehow none of these facts seemed to make me feel better. "How can I write a book about losing weight when half the time I can't even figure out what happened to me or whether it matters or not?" I kept asking my sleepy live-in shrink. He wasn't at his best, and finally, in exhaustion, we both went to sleep.

The next morning when I woke up, Larry was gone. I had slept late, and remembered that he had had an early appointment. Sleepily I wandered into my study. There was a note stuck in my typewriter:

My Dearest Eda,

You ask me what was the use of all you went through to lose weight. You tell me that nothing and no one has changed, that your life is exactly the same as it was before. True, nothing has changed, and yet everything has changed. You have overcome the greatest pain and anguish of your life. You have dealt with your personal demon and stood up to the torment that has always been a part of your existence and finally, once and for all, conquered it.

You will never be the same again. To have done this changes a person. Very few have the courage, the greatness of spirit, to overcome their greatest pain. Those few who do can never, ever, be defeated by life. They carry within them a center of strength and calm that will be with them forever. The finest thing a human being can do—and the hardest task with which we are ever challenged—is to grow past our own special, ultimate inner enemy, the traitor within, and become free of it. Very few ever do this. You did it, and the strength and pride that now belong to you will always be there when you need them. I am terribly proud of knowing you.

All my love,
Larry

When I stopped crying, I knew this beautiful man was right. Everything *has* changed. The daily problems, frustrations and challenges of life will be with me for as long as I live, but in some deep and transcending way I know I cannot ever be defeated. *That* is what it has all been about.

Some months ago Larry told me a story about a man who had climbed one of the highest mountains in the world. He said, "There are two ways to climb a mountain. One way is to simply take a cable car to the summit; the other way is to climb oneself—tearing one's hands on the jagged rocks, learning just where to hang on, to use one's ropes, to deal with slipping and falling, to conquer one's terrors of the always real and present dangers. When one arrives at the top of the mountain, the view is the same whichever way one gets there. *Except that it is not the same at all.*"

I am glad I climbed my special mountain. The view of the world and of myself is my own and indescribably precious. The only thing that really matters is that I did it. I can make no claims on life to reward me for my efforts. The only necessary reward is that I know I did it. It is to that inner center of exultation I invite you—to start climbing your mountain, to conquer your anguish, your enemy within. For no other reason than that forever after, you will know the courage of which you are capable.